Principles and Practices of Complete Dentures

— creating the mental image of a denture —

Iwao Hayakawa D.D.S., D.D.Sc.

Associate Professor, Faculty of Dentistry
Tokyo Medical and Dental University, Tokyo, Japan

Quintessence Publishing Co., Ltd.

Tokyo, Chicago, Berlin, London, Paris, Barcelona, São Paulo, Milano, Copenhagen, Istanbul,

Moscow, Prague, Warsaw and New Delhi

Hayakawa, Iwao
"Principles and Practices of Complete Dentures
— creating the metal image of a denture —"

© 2001 by Quintessence Publishing Co., Ltd. Tokyo
All rights reserved.

Printed in China
ISBN 4-87417-607-0 C3047

Preface

Nowadays, people's lives span over 80 years or more and dental clinics are becoming increasingly crowded with elderly patients. They might be thinking "Life is short, so let's live everyday to its fullest!". Certainly, when considering quality of life, "eating" is just as important as "watching" for elderly people. However, unfortunately very few elderly patients are satisfied with their complete dentures and I hear that many patients have already given up using their dentures.

Even in this situation, many dentists seem to dislike complete denture practice, assuming that it is too difficult. So I have actively written about mainly clinical techniques in journals so as to encourage dentists to maintain an interest in "complete dentures". However, since the working steps such as impression making, jaw registration, teeth arrangement and contouring of the polished surface were written separately, I felt that many points were not clear about the relationships between these steps. When Quintessence Publishing Company asked me to write a book, I felt this was an excellent opportunity to present these relationships, thereby undertaking this task with great pleasure.

A denture has its value only when it functions comfortably and smoothly in the mouth. In writing this book, I have tried to explain how, through "visualization", we can create a "mental image" of the form of the final denture and how this can be related to denture design. In doing so, rather than reviewing the established principles, I have concentrated on the underlying philosophy of complete denture construction. However, I will be very happy if this book enables the reader to construct successful dentures using this underlying philosophy.

Although the technical procedures should not be omitted for sequential explanation, due to limited page space, I have only mentioned those procedures I wished to highlight.

From my experiences of demonstrating the art of origami (paper folding) to my children, I often found the instruction books contained complicated illustrations which even adults could hardly understand. Therefore I have tried to write this book as simply as possible.

After finishing this book, I was not satisfied with some of the contents. I hope I may receive useful suggestions which will enable further revision of this book.

I would like to deeply thank Professor Masanori Nagao, Department of Gerodontology, Tokyo Medical and Dental University, for his invaluable advice. I would also like to thank my former teacher, Emeritus Professor Toshio Hayashi, Tokyo Medical and Dental University, for his worthwhile teachings. Also I appreciate the help from the staff of Quintessence Publishing Company for their editing, Mr. Kazuhide Tuchihira and Mr. Hisashi Matsubara, Department of Dental Technology, Tokyo Medical and Dental University, for their technical procedures. Thanks are also due to Dr. Hiroyuki Uchida and Dr. Eiji Osada, Department of Gerodontology, Tokyo Medical and Dental University, for their helpful assistance with the photographs.

Now that 32 years have passed since I first practiced complete denture prosthodontics, I feel very happy that I was able to spend all those years in research and clinical practice of this profound field. With this edition I would like to express my thanks to my late father, Ryozo Hayakawa, Former Professor of Prosthodontics, Nihon University, for his guidance to live with complete dentures.

Iwao Hayakawa

Contents

Section 4

Arranging the artificial teeth   63

Section 5

Try-in of the dentures   91

Section 6

Designing the polished surface   97

Commentaries

Prologue:
Imaging complete dentures

The size and life span of the elderly population is increasing, but we have not heard that the life span of teeth is increasing. As a result, the period for wearing complete dentures is increasing. For example, a person who has worn a denture for 5 years previously may now live 5 more years, increasing the wearing period, and thus doubling the years of use of the denture. I am afraid that the increased period of denture wearing is causing changes in the alveolar ridges and other tissues around the denture, which we have never previously experienced.

Undoubtedly we are coming across more and more poor alveolar ridges. When ill-fitting dentures are used, an easy case will become a difficult case and a difficult case even more chaotic. From this standpoint, we must preserve the present state of the oral cavity by making suitable dentures. They may minimize the possibility of soft tissue abuse and bone resorption. If we don't make an effort to minimize changes in the mouth, we may start to loose favorable oral conditions neccesary for successful denture design.

In daily practice, we seldom find dentures categorized as complete dentures and often hear that complete denture techniques are difficult.

The techniques of complete denture construction are not so difficult when compared with the high level of manual dexterity required for crown and bridge work where good craftsmanship is of the utmost importance. In complete denture construction, it seems that accumulated knowledge and technical experience are more important. Certainly, with increasing age and poorer vision, the preparation of abutment teeth becomes more difficult. As we become older our experience mounts up more and more and consequently, we become more skilful in denture making and thus we will never be defeated by our sons. However, effective training based on the knowledge of the anatomy and physiology of the tissues and structures that support and surround dentures and materials will give us a

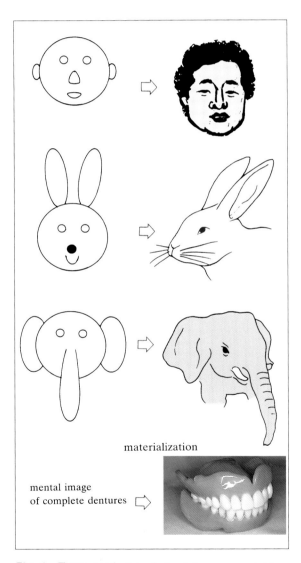

materialization

mental image
of complete dentures ⇨

Fig. 1 Every product is derived from a mental image. Shouldn't you create the mental image of a denture before fabrication?

greater chance of constructing successful dentures.

Regrettably, there are many dentists who lose their interest in complete dentures because of the misconception that complete denture techniques are too difficult. In order that they might gain an interest in complete dentures and acquire the techniques effectively, I have been teaching the complete denture subject from the "form" point of view. I have been pleased to find that young dentists are able to understand the technical procedures much better as a result.

I teach that the form, position and behavior of people's tongues, cheeks and lips are almost all the same, so a denture which is placed between these structures would possess a "form" common to all. Therefore, it is only necessary to learn one general form or concept of complete dentures and then construct a denture just by referring to it. Each denture is a variation of the common form. In denture fabrication, if we can create the mental image of the new complete denture before impression making, the job would be almost finished. The remaining procedures are only to change the image into the form of the denture. In other words, if we know "what form the complete denture should possess?" it would be easier to construct a complete denture successfully(Fig. 1).

We must understand the significance of the anatomy and physiology of the structures which surround dentures in order to create the mental image. It would be helpful to see properly crafted dentures for this purpose. An artist has to see a great many high quality paintings to improve his/her work. Also when learning "igo"(a Japanese game) and "shogi" (Japanese chess), one should find a good teacher to get the chance to see good matches and study advanced techniques. Thus one is able to master the strategy and become a better player more quickly.

By carefully listening to the patient's complaint about the existing denture, we will gain useful information. The denture should be examined and using this information, modified to an improved form close to the final image. This procedure is essential for training to create the image.

Section 1

Examination and preparation for treatment

Examination and preparation for treatment

As most edentulous patients are elderly, the examination must be carried out not only with regard to the condition of the oral cavity, but in relation to their general health. However, sometimes dentists with less clinical experience may reach for an impression tray and start making the impression as soon as the patient sits in the dental chair without a definite treatment plan. If we want to make a successful denture, we must first conduct a thorough extra and intraoral examination of the mouth including the condition of the existing denture, denture-supporting areas, the condition of the temporomandibular joint and the appearance. The intraoral examination, in particular, should be done not only by glancing at, but also by closely observing and palpating the alveolar ridge(Fig. 1-1). For example, if the bone resorption is severe, the alveolar ridges are flattened and moreover the mylohyoid ridge is sharpened on the lingual side and the covering mucosa is very thin. These points can be determined by palpating the areas. If such areas are found, we should think about using relief and a soft lining material(Fig. 1-2).

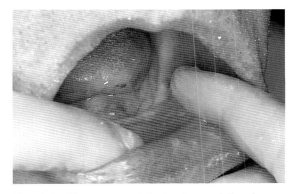

Fig. 1-1 First we must look at, carefully observe and then palpate the alveolar ridge.

1. Surgical treatment

Certain oral conditions require surgical treatment to improve the environment for denture construction. If there is redness or an ulcer over the area where the denture impinges, we can eliminate it by adjusting the denture. If there is widespread inflammation over the denture-bearing mucosa, it will recover quickly by removal of the denture for 2-3 days or by use of a tissue conditioning material. However, surgical treatment is still necessary for the denture-bearing tissues of some edentulous patients. Other cases may only require rehabilitation by prosthodontic means, but surgical modification is sometimes advantageous to improve the retention and stability of the denture.

The wearing of an ill-fitting denture for a long time causes

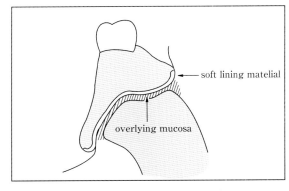

Fig. 1-2 In the case of severe alveolar bone resorption, palpation is inevitable. If spiny ridges and thin covering mucosa are felt, we have to think about relief and soft liners.

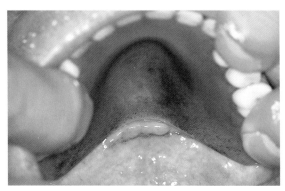

Fig. 1-3   A so-called denture fibroma caused by repeated irritation due to prolonged wearing of an ill-fitting denture.

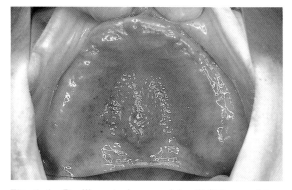

Fig. 1-4   Papillomatosis caused by ill-fitting and improperly cleaned dentures.

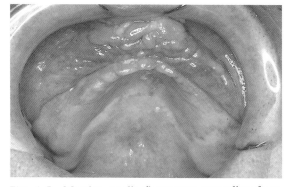

Fig. 1-5   Massive epulis fissuratum extending from the anterior residual ridge to the oral vestibule under an ill-fitting denture. Surgical treatment is inevitable.

repeated irritation to the mucosa during chewing, and consequently fibrous growth of the tissue will occur as a defense response. Soft tissue hyperplasia occurs under or around a complete denture and is referred to as so-called flabby gums or denture fibroma(Fig. 1-3). As flabby gums, which are seen in the anterior residual ridge of the maxilla and mandible, are highly compressible and displaceable, it is difficult to make an impression in the usual way. When this is not excessive, a good result may be possible by proper prosthodontic treatment, but a severe case may need surgical intervention. Elderly people may have difficulty in cleaning their dentures and mouth sufficiently and thus the prolonged wearing of an ill-fitting denture might lead to a stomatitis like papillomatosis(Fig. 1-4). In mild cases, healing may occur after resting the tissues which can be achieved by removal of the dentures and improvement of oral hygiene.

In certain cases, it is impossible to make impressions without any surgical treatment. Figure 1-5 shows a so-called denture fibroma. A massive roll of hyperplastic tissue which extends from the anterior residual ridge to the oral vestibule in the maxilla is referred to as epulis fissuratum and needs to be excised surgically before making a new denture. However, when we eliminate a wide area as in this case, if we try to eliminate all the pathological tissue, it may leave a scar in the area which is essential for denture retention and consequently, the subsequent prosthodontic treatment will become harder. So, we must decide the area of elimination by careful treatment planning which will be favorable for further procedures(Fig. 1-6).

Some cases have large undercuts in the region of the tuberosity or anterior residual ridges. If the flanges in these areas are extended deep into the sulci for the peripheral seal, these undercuts might interfere with denture insertion and removal. When there is an undercut on only one side, the insertion of the denture is possible by rotating it into position and this undercut may even enhance denture retention(Fig. 1-7). However, when there are undercuts on both sides, surgical elimination or easing of the denture border must be performed. In the case of surgical treatment, it is important that the amount of bone removed should be as minimal as possible because many undercuts are covered by compressible mucosa and are not as large as we expect.

The other indications for pre-prosthetic surgery are a pendulous maxillary tuberosity, prominent maxillary torus and mandibular tori, excessive undercuts, spiny ridges, etc. In cases with severe alveolar bone resorption where the denture-supporting tissues are limited, surgical procedures such as vestibuloplasty or ridge augmentation may be carried out.

Although surgical treatments may be necessary for a good result, for elderly patients, the physical and mental trauma might effect their general health and therefore surgical treatment is sometimes better avoided. Even if they can withstand the surgery, in advanced age, the healing processes are delayed and post-operative conditions of the oral cavity may be more severe.

In any case, the indiscriminate use of surgery just for prosthodontic convenience should be avoided. Surgery should be avoided if at all possible and the denture should be improved by various prosthodontic techniques such as varying the impression technique and providing appropriate relief over the affected area.

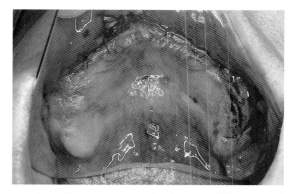

Fig. 1-6 The area of elimination should be decided after careful planning. In the case of Fig. 1-5 the flabby gums of the anterior region were left, as prosthodontic means could be performed. Minimizing the area of the elimination produced a good result.

2. Correcting the occlusion

It is important to examine whether any problems of the temporomandibular joint may be present and also the occlusion of the existing dentures. A patient wearing ill-fitting dentures for a long time tends to occlude in a position far away from the centric occlusal position as a result of the functional adaptation in which one masticates in a position comfortable to him/herself. This is the so-called "habitual bite" and will cause a decrease in masticatory efficiency and moreover lead to mandibular dysfunction.

The habitual eccentric occlusion should be treated before making new dentures. However, because the muscles of mastication have learned the habitual eccentric jaw position for a long time, sudden correction is not easy. Generally, the habi-

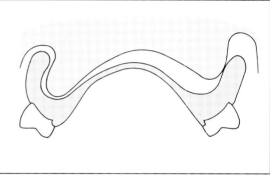

Fig. 1-7 When there is a unilateral undercut, the denture can be inserted and removed by rotating it into position. It will even enhance denture retention.

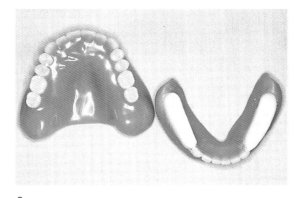

a

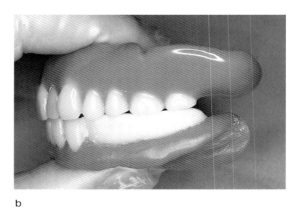

b

Fig. 1-8a,b The flattened occlusal surface eliminates the intercuspation of the artificial teeth in the habitual eccentric jaw position and therefore can relieve the stiffness in the muscles and joints. Without the limitation of the cusps, the jaw can gradually return to its centric occlusal position.

tual eccentric occlusion may be corrected by wearing treatment dentures for a relatively long period of time. The patient will also be satisfied with the recovery of the occlusion by treatment dentures and further recording of the maxillomandibular relationship will be smooth and accurate(Fig. 8a,b).

3. Flow of saliva

Through aging, salivary flow decreases and its contents change. As saliva enhances denture retention by intervening between the denture and the mucosa, a patient with scanty saliva will have poor denture retention. Also in a dry oral cavity, the mucosa lying beneath the denture base may be easily traumatized and therefore the impression surface of the denture must be polished more smoothly. The diminution in salivary flow will not moisten the oral mucosa and will interfere with the functions of mastication, swallowing and phonetics. In some cases, the use of artificial saliva or medications promoting salivary secretion should be recommended.

4. Patient's requests and desires

There is one more important step in the examination. At the patient's first visit to the clinic, we must quickly and precisely gather what (s)he requests mostly from his/her complaints about the existing dentures. Their requests might be confined to mastication, esthetics or phonetics.

It once happened that a patient repeatedly came to my clinic and complained of pain, even though the dentures were thought to be perfect and no ulcers or inflammation could be found on the mucosa. Finally, it was proved that the patient's complaint was not pain, but the appearance of the arrangement of the anterior teeth. If the patient is satisfied with the appearance, (s)he would definitely wear the denture even with a little bit of pain or a poor fit. Complaints related to esthetics are difficult to find as the patient is sometimes too embarrassed to talk about them and sometimes it is even an underlying complaint which the patient is not conscious of. Therefore a careful examination which involves gathering the patient's requests is recommended.

In any case, the denture is a piece of work constructed by the dentist, but the patient becomes its owner after insertion. We can be no more proud of, or satisfied with, our dentures as wonderful products by ourselves alone. It is important to make the denture suit the patient so that the new dentures can truly become his/her own. For this, we must make a denture that contains the patient's "heart". The denture should never be a "stranger" to the patient. In other words, only when the patient's requests have been included in the denture, will it then become his/her own denture. The complaints of the patient are often unclear, misunderstood and confused; however, I believe that they have expressed their honest feelings and I have therefore tried to listen to their words carefully.

Section 2

Making the impressions

Making the impressions

In a favorable denture case where alveolar bone resorption is minimal and the cross section of the alveolar ridge resembles a U-shaped outline, border molding during impression making is easy. A proper impression is made possible just by reproducing the contour of the sulcus onto the impression as it is seen. However, in an unfavorable case with severe alveolar bone resorption due to severe periodontitis or prolonged wearing of an ill-fitting denture, some dentists might be puzzled how to take the impression and how to extend the denture borders correctly. In these unfavorable cases, if the denture border is placed at the junction of immovable gingivae and movable mucosa only by passive hand manipulations, it will result in the so-called cord-like denture, leading to poor denture retention, especially in the mandible.

As is generally known, the wider the denture base area, the better the denture retention will be. Therefore the impression making — not impression taking — should be performed actively according to our objectives so that the denture base area can be enlarged as much as possible. However, it is not appropriate to extend the denture border at random. The denture border should be appropriately extended in the areas where it is possible to extend it and the border should be limited where extention is not required. In order to perform this, initially it is important to understand what form the denture base should take and then the impression making is carried out in accordance with that mental image.

When the condition of the alveolar ridge is unfavorable, some dentists may say, "Only after impression taking can the situation of the alveolar ridge be grasped or the denture border can be shaped". However, if we are not convinced of the contour of the impression before impression making, we will never obtain a successful denture. It is like admitting defeat before beginning the battle.

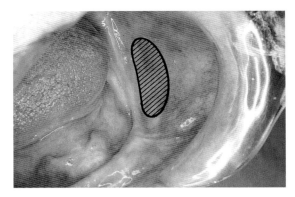

Fig. 2-1 In the flat ridge, the area for resistance to occlusal forces would depend on the buccal shelf. It is bounded medially by the alveolar crest, anteriorly by the buccal frenum, laterally by the external oblique ridge and distally by the retromolar pad.

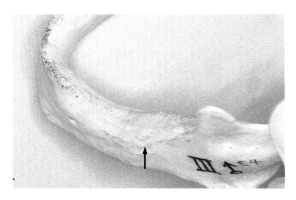

Fig. 2-2 Outside the buccal shelf, a ridge runs anteroposteriorly which is called the external oblique ridge. It is not involved in resorption.

1. Landmarks for the mandibular impression

Buccal flange area

In the poor situation where the ridges are flat and the movable mucosa reaches up to the crest of the alveolar ridges, the sole area of resistance to occlusal forces would be the buccal shelf which is situated on the buccal side of the area of the posterior teeth. The buccal shelf is covered with dense cortical bone and is also a wide area lying perpendicular to the direction of the occlusal forces. Therefore, it is an appropriate area for denture support(Fig. 2-1). Thus, in severely resorbed ridges, there must be no doubt in using the buccal shelf as the denture support. The buccal shelf must be recorded during the impression procedure, otherwise a satisfactory impression will not result.

Outside the buccal shelf, a bony ridge runs anteroposteriorly which is called the external oblique ridge and is used as a landmark for the denture border. The denture border can be extended 1-2 mm beyond the external oblique ridge and therefore the ridge must be recorded by making the impression(Fig. 2-2,3,4).

However, if the denture border is extended beyond the external oblique ridge, the denture base will be widened over the buccinator muscle attachment and thus located on the buccinator muscle fibers(Fig. 2-5).

On the buccal shelf, the buccinator muscle fibers run close to the bone, and are thin, tendinous and thus inactive. In addition, the lower muscle bundles of the buccinator are not tense and slacken laterally from the external oblique ridge

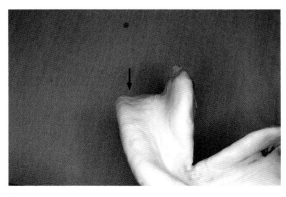

Fig. 2-3 In the impression, the external oblique ridge shows a groove. The impression should record the ridge. The denture border can be extended 1-2 mm beyond this ridge.

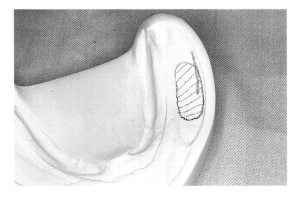

Fig. 2-4 The buccal shelf is a wide area lying perpendicular to the direction of occlusal force and is therefore an appropriate area for denture support.

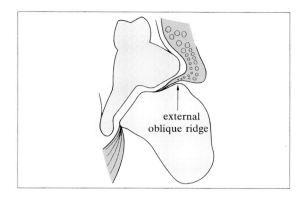

Fig. 2-5 If the denture border is extended beyond the external oblique ridge, the denture base will cover the buccinator muscle fibers. However, since the lower muscle bundle of the buccinator is loose and inactive, it will not dislodge the denture.

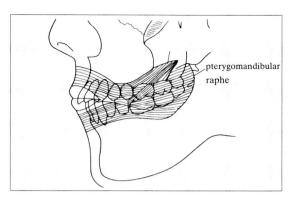

Fig. 2-6 The fibers of the buccinator run anteroposteriorly, so that the force dislodging the denture during mastication is minimal(Illustration from Kamijo, Y.).

area. The muscle fibers run anteroposteriorly, paralleling the denture border and function in a horizontal direction. Therefore, the force dislodging the denture during mastication is small and thus it is possible to extend the denture border into this area(Fig. 2-6).

If the denture border is underextended in this area, it is difficult to mould the convex buccal flange correctly(P. 104), leading to food accumulation in the buccal sulcus and under the denture base(Fig. 2-7).

Mylohyoid ridge area

If the denture border is short of the mylohyoid ridge, it will dig into the residual ridge and cause pain. The border is shortened to remove this pain, but shortly after, the shortened border again impinges upon the residual ridge. Finally this repetition will make the denture into a cord-like denture which has poorer retention and stability(Fig. 2-8, 9).

Border molding of the mylohyoid ridge area should be performed to cover the ridge 4-6 mm beyond it. At the insertion appointment, the impression surface of the denture on the mylohyoid ridge is relieved so that pain during mastication will be diminished(Fig. 2-10).

In addition, when the lingual denture border is extended properly as mentioned above, the lingual polished surface can be shaped into a concave form(the concave shelf, P.103) which is important for the retention and stability of the denture(Fig. 2-11).

In a serious case where the residual ridge is poor, the membranous attachment of the floor of the mouth appears high in the mylohyoid area. This appearance may lead dentists to assume that the muscles are strained parallel to the floor of

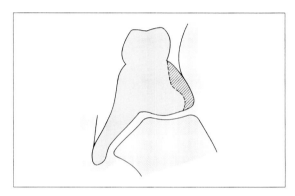

Fig. 2-7 If the denture border is underextended in the buccal shelf area, a convex buccal flange will not be possible, so it will not be able to occupy the buccal pouch. A space will occur between the denture border and the lower muscle bundle of the buccinator, resulting in food accumulation.

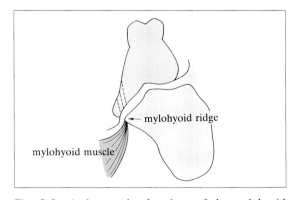

Fig. 2-8 A denture border short of the mylohyoid ridge digs into the residual ridge and causes pain. If shortened, the denture border will impinge again upon the ridge.

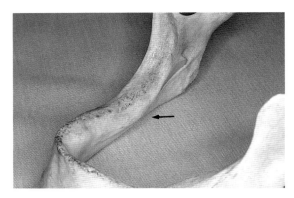

Fig. 2-9 In severe alveolar ridge resorption, the mylohyoid ridge becomes prominent and causes pain when pressure is applied by the denture.

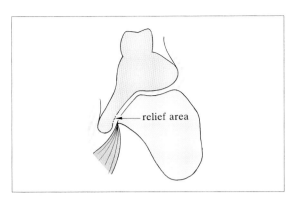

Fig. 2-10 Border molding of the mylohyoid ridge area should be performed 4-6 mm below this ridge. Later the impression surface of the denture on the mylohyoid ridge area is relieved.

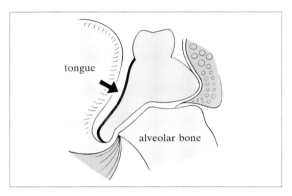

Fig. 2-11 The properly extended lingual flange can be shaped into a "concave shelf"(thickened line), which is useful for retention and stability of the denture.

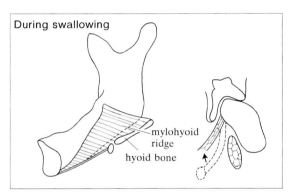

Fig. 2-12 As the mylohyoid muscle runs anteroinferiorly even when it contracts maximally, it allows extension of the denture border beyond the mylohyoid ridge(Modified from Kamijo, Y.).

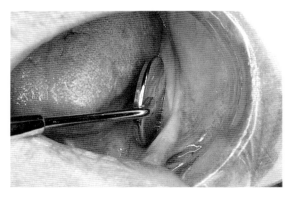

Fig. 2-13 Testing the tension forces with a finger or a mouth mirror.

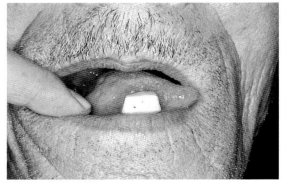

Fig. 2-14 Exaggerated tongue movement in which the tongue is protruded outside the dental arch to record the mylohyoid muscle during impression taking.

the mouth during contraction which might cause pain or denture dislodgment and therefore the denture borders tend to be mistakenly shortened. However, as the muscle fibers run anteroinferiorly even during maximum muscle contraction, it is possible to extend the denture border beyond the mylohyoid ridge to which the mylohyoid muscle attaches(Fig. 2-12). Moreover, in the case of the elderly, the contraction of the mylohyoid muscle is not so strong. The muscle tension can be evaluated by palpating the floor of the mouth with a finger or a mouth mirror(Fig. 2-13).

When making an impression of this region, some think that the movement of the mylohyoid muscle would be recorded by moving the tip of tongue toward the opposite side. However, tongue movement is due to the action of the genioglossus muscle(Fig. 2-14). The mylohyoid muscle contracts during swallowing. By this tongue movement, instead of the movement of the mylohyoid muscle, the movement of the floor of the mouth which might be strained by the tongue will be recorded. This movement of the tongue can be considered to be exaggerated.

As exaggerated tongue movements during impression making will be the cause of underextended borders, excessive movements should be avoided. If the tongue is protruded over the dental arch, the lingual sulcus will become shallow and an extremely shortened border will be obtained. During ordinary functions like mastication, the tongue is never protruded outside the dental arch, like a child's playful gesture of sticking out his/her tongue. If protruded, it might be bitten during mastication. A functional situation is, in other words, not a state of exaggerated movements. Furthermore, even if the dentist understands the tongue movements, during impression taking, it is impossible to expect an elderly patient to follow such a complicated instruction(Fig. 2-15a, b). Impression making should be performed only by the dentist him/herself. It should never be a task requiring assistance from the patient.

As the denture is used in a closed mouth, the tongue should not be moved around too much during impression making. The author never invites tongue movement during impression making. The patient is asked only to relax the tongue comfortably. The impression is then made 4-6 mm below the landmark, the mylohyoid ridge, and thus the extent of the denture border is decided at the mylohyoid ridge area(Fig. 2-16). Even though the case may be favorable for more inferior extension of the border, the border is limited only to this length by trimming the extended border. Of course, denture retention and stability may be better with the lengthened border.

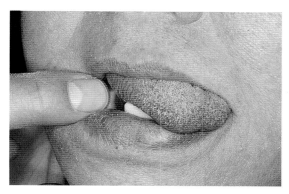

a

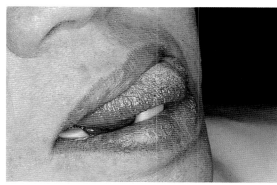

b

Fig. 2-15 The patient is instructed to slightly touch the corner of the mouth with the tongue. The word "slightly" is quite vague and elderly patients can not perform a complicated instruction.

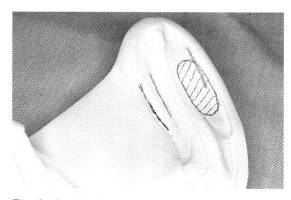

Fig. 2-16 The impression should be made to cover 4-6 mm beyond the mylohyoid ridge. This is the length of the denture border in the mylohyoid ridge area.

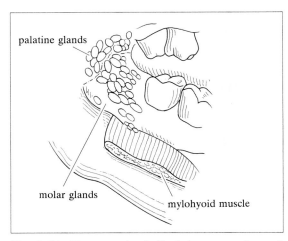

Fig. 2-17 The posterior half of the retromolar pad is filled with resilient glandular tissues(Illustration from Kamijo, Y.). The peripheral seal of the denture can be obtained when the denture border is placed on this tissue.

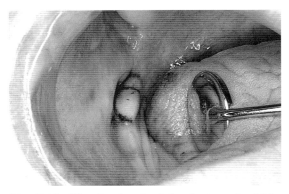

Fig. 2-18 The distal end of the denture should be placed at a point 2/3 of the way up the retromolar pad.

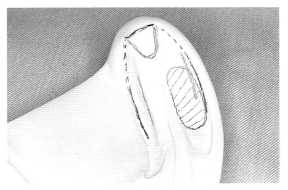

Fig. 2-19 By connecting(dotted lines) the index lines on the buccal side, the distal end and the lingual side, the posterior outline of the denture base can be determined automatically and easily.

However, some patients will complain of tightness at the base of the tongue in lengthened cases. Therefore the denture border should be extended only as far as necessary.

Retromolar pad area

The denture must cover more than half of the retromolar pad. Histologically, the retromolar pad is composed of a firm fibrous connective tissue papilla in its anterior half and soft tissue containing molar glands in the posterior half. These two parts are named separately as the anterior "pear-shaped pad" and the posterior "retromolar pad".[1,2] However, in edentulous cases, it is hard to distinguish them with the naked eye and thus clinically the two parts should be regarded together as the retromolar pad.

The posterior peripheral seal can be obtained by placing the denture border over this resilient glandular tissue(Fig. 2-17). Anywhere is possible on the glandular tissue, but if the denture border is placed too far posteriorly, some patients will complain of tightness at the base of the tongue and therefore it is best to cover 2/3 of the retromolar pad(Fig. 2-18).

As the temporalis muscle fibers attach to the distal portion of the retromolar pad, stimulation from this muscle prevents the pad from resorbing. So, the retromolar pad is also used as a landmark for orientation of the occlusal plane. Therefore the retromolar pad must be included in the impression.

Even though the mandibular molar region is thought to be the most difficult area for impression making, the outline of the denture base can be determined easily and automatically by using these indexes. It is just necessary to connect the index lines, namely lines placed 1 mm beyond the external oblique ridge, 2/3 of the way from the anterior border of the retromolar pad and 4 to 6 mm below the mylohyoid ridge(Fig. 2-19).

However, pain may occur on the buccal side of the retromolar pad region during mastication even though the denture is designed in the above mentioned ways. This is due to the masseter muscle, a strong elevator, which is lateral to the retromolar pad and covers the buccinator muscle. When the masseter muscle contracts, its enlargement presses the denture border with the cramped buccinator muscle. As the denture occludes, it can not move during function of the elevators. So, when the distobuccal border of the denture base is extended into the functioning area of the masseter muscle, the mucosa will be pressed against the denture base leading to pain (Fig. 2-20).

In order to avoid such a situation, the movement of the

masseter muscle is recorded in the impression by creating its reactive contraction through pushing the tray during the border molding procedure. The tension of the masseter muscle will make a concavity in the distobuccal outline of the impression. Another way is to reduce the overlengthened border through observing the redness or displacement of the denture after insertion of the new denture made by connecting the index lines. This method is easier for those who are not familiar with the previous one.

Retromylohyoid fossa

The posterior border of the lingual flange can be the curve obtained by connecting the index lines placed 4-6 mm lower than the mylohyoid ridge and on the retromolar pad. However, it is generally assumed that the denture border lengthened posteroinferiorly into the retromylohyoid fossa can promote retention and stability of the denture(Fig. 2-21). The author has occasionally lengthened the border for those cases with severe bone resorption. However, it has caused the complaint of tightness at the base of the tongue. Therefore retention and stability have been obtained by other means(P. 103) rather than a lengthened border in the majority of cases.

Actually it is very difficult to make a definitive border, namely to make an appropriate impression, in this area. If the denture border is lengthened inappropriately, this will be the worst possible situation and will result in the opposite effect of the aim such as the dislodgment of the denture or an ulcer occurring along the overextended border. The posterior border established by connecting the index lines, as mentioned before, is just enough in cases where retention and stability can be obtained by other means. In almost all cases, the border obtained by this method will be usable. Simplicity is best.

Although the above method is recommended, one may make use of the retromylohyoid fossa.

The space distal to the mylohyoid muscle is referred to as the retromylohyoid fossa. It is bounded by the mylohyoid muscle anteriorly, the retromolar pad laterally, the superior constrictor muscle posterolaterally, the palatoglossus muscle posteromedially, and the tongue medially. There is no structure and so it is possible to lengthen the denture border into this space. During border molding, the border in this area is pushed into the retromylohyoid fossa by the strong intrinsic and extrinsic tongue muscles, and thus it will show the so-called S-curve as viewed from the impression surface(Fig. 2-22). At this time, the posterior limit of the lingual border is defined by the palatoglossus muscle and the lingual slip of the superior constrictor muscle. This is called the retromylohyoid

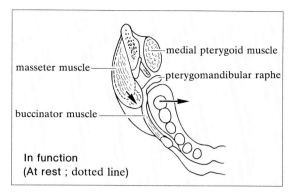

Fig. 2-20 The masseter muscle attaches at the external side of the retromolar pad and covers the buccinator. It indirectly presses the denture border through the cramped buccinator during function(Modified from Kamijo, Y.).

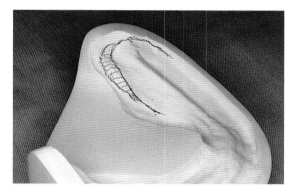

Fig. 2-21 The posterior border of the lingual flange is thought to be lengthened posteroinferiorly in order to obtain retention and stability. However, making the impression in this area is difficult and so the retention and stability should be left to other means.

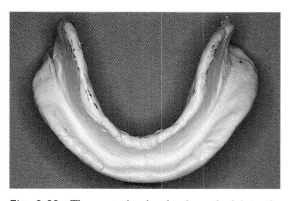

Fig. 2-22 The posterior border is pushed into the fossa by the strong intrinsic and extrinsic tongue muscles, and thus the lingual border of the impression will show the so-called 'S-curve' as viewed from the impression surface.

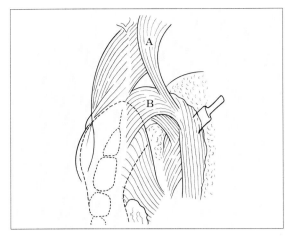

Fig. 2-23 The definitive posterior border of the lingual flange is limited by the palatoglossus muscle, A and the lingual slip of the superior constrictor muscle, B(From Fish, E.W.). This is called the retromylohyoid curtain.

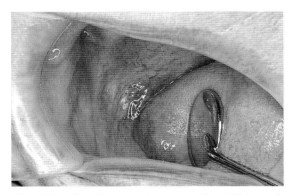

Fig. 2-24 In this case, the retromylohyoid fossa is small and thus it is difficult to extend the denture border.

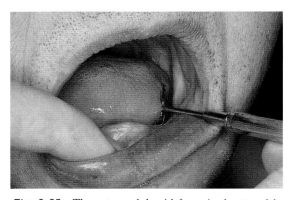

Fig. 2-25 The retromylohyoid fossa is shortened by protrusion of the tongue. The extension area should be evaluated by a mouth mirror when the patient is instructed to make moderate tongue movements.

curtain(Fig. 2-23). When the tongue is protruded, the curtain also moves anteriorly. In some cases, the retromylohyoid fossa becomes greatly shortened and it seems impossible to extend the denture border. The extension of the denture border can be determined by examining the tightness of the fossa with a mouth mirror when the patient is instructed to make moderate tongue movements such as touching the maxillary anterior ridge with the tip of the tongue. Usually the space is wider than expected(Fig. 2-24,25).

By extending the denture flange into this region, a peripheral seal can be obtained continuously from the retromolar pad region to the anterior lingual sulcus. In addition, this extended lingual flange can be shaped accordingly for guiding tongue placement onto the polished surface of the lingual flange. Moreover, the projected posterior border will literally serve as a flange(the projecting edge of a train wheel) by physical means, leading to an improved denture.[3,4]

Sublingual gland area

The sublingual gland lies above the mylohyoid muscle. The gland is raised when the mylohyoid muscle contracts during swallowing(Fig. 2-26). The position of the mucosa of the floor of the mouth may be recorded higher through impression making by excessively moving the tip of the tongue. However, the lingual flange extension is decreased and a space is created between the denture border and the mucosa of the floor of the mouth whilst the mylohyoid muscle is at rest, leading to impairment of the peripheral seal(Fig. 2-27).

Similar to impression making in the mylohyoid ridge area, the patient is never instructed to perform any movements of the tongue, but asked only to relax the tongue comfortably. The mouth is nearly closed and the tongue lies on the floor of the mouth completely. This is the "impression position" of the tongue(Fig. 2-28). Through border molding, the depth of the lingual vestibule is recorded in this situation and this will in turn be used as the length of the lingual flange in the sublingual gland area, so that the lingual border seal can be established effectively(Fig. 2-29).

Is this length all right when the sublingual gland is raised by the contracted mylohyoid muscle or not?

The lower denture will not be lifted up, even though the sublingual gland is raised, as the upper and lower teeth are in contact when swallowing. On the other hand, the sublingual gland serves as a cushion due to its soft and resilient nature and therefore it will neither lift the denture nor will its covering mucosa be traumatized by the denture(Fig. 2-30). This length is quite enough for normal functional movements.

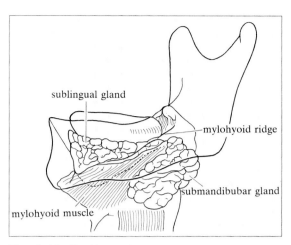

Fig. 2-26 Position of the sublingual gland(From Kamijo, Y.). It lies above the mylohyoid muscle and is raised by the contracted mylohyoid during swallowing.

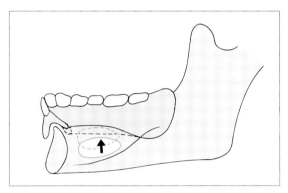

Fig. 2-27 If the denture border is made short to relieve the raised sublingual gland, a space will occur between the denture border and the mucosa when the mylohyoid muscle is at rest and thus the peripheral seal will be lost.

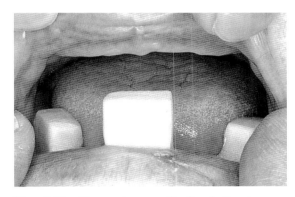

Fig. 2-28 "Impression position" of the tongue. Complicated instructions are never given to the patient. The patient is asked just to relax the tongue comfortably.

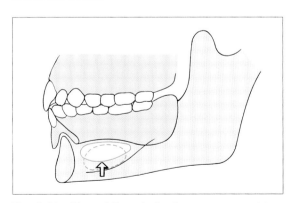

Fig. 2-30 The sublingual gland serves as a cushion, so neither lifts the denture nor causes the mucosa to be traumatized by the denture.

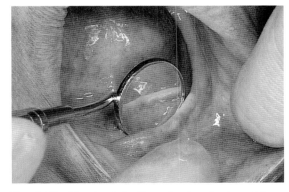

Fig. 2-29 Depth of the lingual sulcus in the sublingual gland area is recorded when the tongue is relaxed.

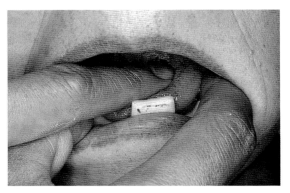

Fig. 2-31   Tongue movements are made by pressing the anterior portion of the tongue with the forefinger. Such an amount of tongue movement is recommended for those who want to make tongue movements.

Retruded tongue position

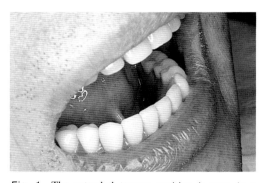

Fig. 1   The retruded tongue position is seen in a slightly opened mouth. This is found in 25% of people. It is hard to maintain the lingual peripheral seal, and thus air or food easily enter beneath the lingual borders.

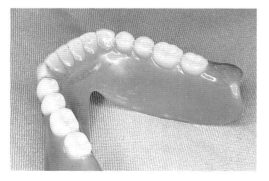

Fig. 2   Retruded tongue position can be corrected by having patients train themselves to place their tongue over the groove on the lingual surface of the denture.

In a slightly opened mouth, the tongue appears relaxed and completely covers the floor of the mouth with the tip of the tongue lightly contacting the lingual surfaces of the lower anterior teeth and the lateral border of the tongue covering the occlusal surfaces of the posterior teeth. This is the normal position of the tongue[5]. This tongue position is quite favorable for maintaining the lingual peripheral seal which improves retention and stability of the denture.

However, such a normal tongue position is missing in some people. Wright et al.[6] found that about 75% of people had a normal tongue position, but the remaining had a retruded tongue position. In these cases, it is hard to obtain a peripheral seal as air or food can easily enter beneath the lingual borders(Fig. 1). Even the "concave shelf", as mentioned later, can not work effectively.

It is thought that the retruded tongue position can be improved by training the tongue. Levin reported that the following method proved successful for many patients[7].

A small "training groove" about 10 mm long, 2 mm wide, and 2 mm deep is made just below the central incisors(Fig. 2). The patient is instructed to place the tongue on the groove at all times except when eating and speaking. The edges of the groove are slightly tapered and smooth so as not to irritate the tongue. He reported that most patients could learn to keep the tongue on this correct position within a few weeks. Finally, the training groove is filled with auto-polymerizing acrylic resin.

However, it must be noted not to insert the tray carelessly because the patient might open his/her mouth widely and roll up the tongue.

Some dentists are not satisfied unless tongue movements are used to record the movement of the floor of the mouth. The movements should be carried out by pressing the anterior portion of the tongue with the forefinger of the operator's other hand during impression making. Only such an degree of tongue movement is recommended(Fig. 2-31). Exaggerated tongue movements will cause an underextended denture border.

Labial flange area

The orbicularis oris is the major muscle in this region. As its muscle fibers run horizontally, care must be taken not to overextend the impression border in cases with weak muscle tension in this region.

The mentalis muscle is one of the muscles constituting the lower lip. Its muscle fibers are vertical and the origin attaches high on the mandibular alveolar process, therefore the labial vestibule becomes shallow when this muscle contracts. However, if the lip is pulled too much as a result of being over conscious about this contraction during border molding, the vestibule will become too shallow because the attachment of the muscle is higher than the base of the labial vestibule(Fig. 2-33).

In patients exhibiting strong muscle tension of these muscles in this region, this causes the lower lip to fall inwards and the impression border becomes thin and short. As a result, the completed denture might have an insufficient peripheral seal. In general, the instruction is given to bite the operator's fingers which are placed between the tray and the maxillary ridge. As the masticatory muscles become tense and the lower lip becomes loose as a reflex, the impression is then made in this situation(Fig. 2-34).

Usually it is recommended that the patient is instructed to close the mouth slightly with relaxed lips and the lower lip is pulled lightly outwards and the depth of the vestibule is recorded as it is seen(Fig. 2-35). However, with this method a portion of the mentalis muscle will be covered by the denture base. So care should be taken not to apply excessive pressure with the insufficiently softened compound during border molding and moreover, the impression surface of the completed denture should be carefully adjusted using pressure-indicating paste. In the case of severe ridge resorption, it may be difficult to recognize the inferior labial frenum even though the lower lip is pulled outwards. It need not be recorded forc-

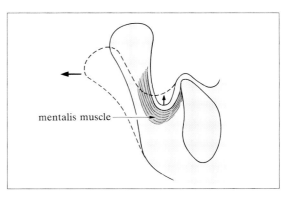

Fig. 2-33 When the lip is pulled too much during border molding, the vestibule becomes shallow as the mentalis muscle attachment is higher than the base of the labial vestibule.

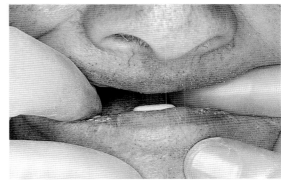

Fig. 2-34 On biting the operator's fingers, the masticatory muscles become tense and the lips become relaxed as a reflex, then the impression is made in this situation.

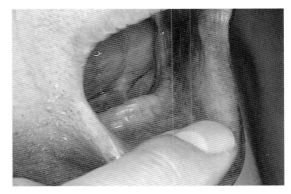

Fig. 2-35 The lip is pulled lightly outwards and the depth of the labial vestibule is recorded as it is seen.

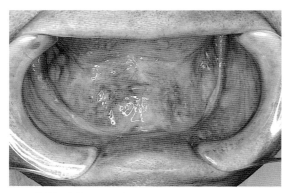

Fig. 2-36   The genial tubercles are the origins of both the genioglossus and geniohyoid muscles. They do not undergo bone resorption. They can project prominently in cases of severe bone resorption.

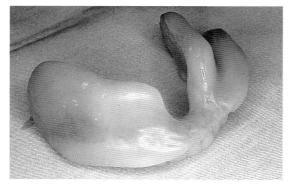

Fig. 2-37   The denture flange is widely eliminated in the genial tubercles region in many dentures for fear that this part may be loaded when the denture moves tissueward due to occlusal forces.(This is the denture of the patient shown in Fig. 2-36, which has been lined with a tissue conditioner by the patient himself to avoid movement of the denture.)

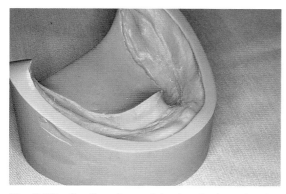

Fig. 2-38   Confirm the genial tubercles by palpation and then try to cover them with the denture. The peripheral seal can never be established when the denture border ends on hard tissues.(the case of Fig. 2-36)

ibly, but if the frenum is irritated by the completed denture, relief should be provided.

Anterior lingual flange area

The border of the impression in this area is mainly influenced by the lingual frenum and the genioglossus muscle. Sometimes the lingual frenum is broad. The strong genioglossus muscle lies just beneath the lingual frenum and its action is mainly to raise and protrude the tongue.

The genial tubercles, which are the origins of both the genioglossus muscle and the geniohyoid muscle, are hardly involved in the process of alveolar bone resorption. Thus in the case of severe bone resorption, the genial tubercles project higher than the crest of the residual ridge. The projection is extremely prominent in some cases(Fig. 2-36).

The denture flange covering the genial tubercles may be widely eliminated in many dentures for fear that the tubercles would be irritated by settling of the denture due to occlusal forces(Fig. 2-37). However, if the denture border ends on the hard tissues, no peripheral seal will be possible. The denture border must be extended over the genial tubercles in favor of improving the peripheral seal(Fig. 2-38, 39).

The genioglossus muscle and the lingual frenum which lies over the muscle move actively and are easily traumatized, therefore their movements and tension must be recorded exactly during border molding. Thus the patient must be instructed to make appropriate tongue movements in order to record the exact depth and width of the notch made by the lingual frenum. To provide adequate clearance in this area, the patient is instructed to make some overactive movements such as licking the lower lip by moving the tip of the tongue from side to side. Inadequate clearance may result in pain or

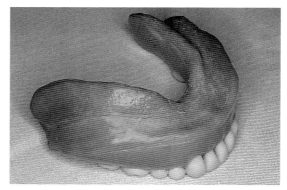

Fig. 2-39   The denture border covers the genial tubercles for the peripheral seal.(This is a new denture for the case in Fig. 2-36 which has been lined with a soft liner.)

inflammation. Tongue movement is never requested during impression making. However, this is the only area where functional movement of the tongue is necessary. But this procedure may require great skill. If the clearance is too wide, the denture will loose its seal, which is important for retention. Finally the denture should be trimmed little by little by properly examining the denture after it has been inserted.

The internal surface of the denture covering the genial tubercles should be adjusted carefully using pressure-indicating paste at the time of denture insertion. Therefore appropriate relief on the impression, or fitting surface of the denture base is provided, which compensates for the amount of tissueward movement of the denture resulting from occlusal forces.

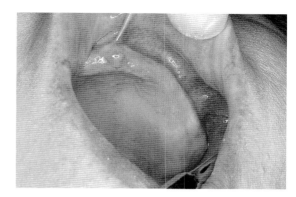

Fig. 2-40 The length of the border should be recorded as deeply as the sulcus is observed.

2. Landmarks for the maxillary impression

Maxillary border molding is easier than that for the mandible except for those cases with a flat ridge and little or no vestibular space. The length of the border will be adequate if the sulcus is recorded as deeply as it is observed(Fig. 2-40). Even if the length of the border is inadequate, it is thought that good retention is possible by the so-called 'facial seal' which is created by the drape of the lips and cheeks[7]. Thus, the only areas where care is needed in impression making for the maxillary denture are the frenal, buccal vestibular, and posterior border areas.

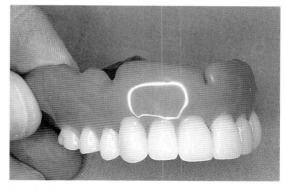

Fig. 2-41 The labial notch is long and narrow. The buccal notch is wide and V-shaped.

Frenal area

The maxillary labial frenum is a fold of mucous membrane mainly consisting of fibrous connective tissue. It tenses between the labial gingiva and the upper lip mucosa when the upper lip is raised. A labial notch is formed in the denture border due to the movement of this frenum.

The lip movement near the maxillary labial frenum is vertical and thus the notch becomes long and narrow. If the frenum is pulled too far laterally during border molding, the notch will become too wide and the peripheral seal will be lost, therefore care is needed so as not to manipulate the lip excessively (Fig. 2-41).

In some cases, depressions are recorded beside the labial frenum notch due to muscle bands consisting of the origins of the nasal septal depressor muscle and the orbicularis oris[5]. In these cases, the denture must be adequately relieved so as not to disturb the function of these muscles.

On the other hand, the muscle movements around the buccal frenum are both vertical and horizontal, thus a wider

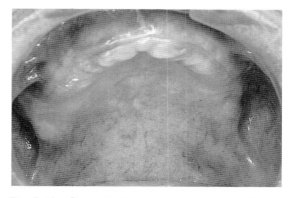

Fig. 2-42 Generally the buccal frenum runs obliquely in a posterior direction, and so its anterior movement should be recorded by pursing the lips.

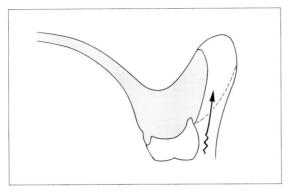

Fig. 2-43 If border molding in the buccal space is inadequate, the denture will lose its seal because of the ingress of air under the denture base when the buccal vestibule is opened during situations in which the patient laughs and opens the mouth widely.

notch should be formed compared with the labial frenum. It will become a V-shaped notch. Generally the frenum runs obliquely and posteriorly, therefore its anterior movement should be recorded by pursing the lips such as when whistling, during border molding(Fig. 2-42).

Buccal vestibular area

The vestibule which extends posteriorly from the buccal frenum, the so-called the buccal space, should be recorded just as it is seen. Even though it appears rather wide, the impression should be made as it is seen. If this space is inadequately formed, the denture will lose its peripheral seal because of the ingress of air under the denture base due to the opening up of the buccal vestibule when the patient laughs and opens the mouth widely(Fig. 2-43, 44a~d). In addition, it may not lead to an appropriate arrangement of artificial teeth and a proper polished surface(P. 84, The importance of the impression of the buccal space).

In the rare case when it is hard to determine the width of

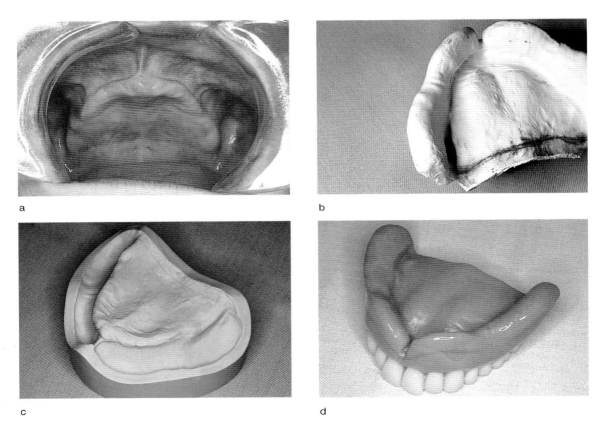

a

b

c

d

Fig. 2-44a~d In a severely resorbed ridge the vestibule appears rather wide, but it should be recorded as it is seen without any hesitation. An adequately widened impression will lead to an appropriate arrangement of artificial teeth and a proper polished surface.

the vestibule and thus the width of the denture border, due to severe alveolar ridge resorption(Fig. 2-45), the appropriate width of the vestibule can be estimated by using the remnants of the lingual gingival margin as a guide.

Watt measured the buccolingual breadth of the dentate alveolar ridge(the horizontal breadth of the alveolar process from the lingual gingival margin to the maximal projection of the buccal surface of the ridge) and found that this measurement for every tooth position was remarkably constant. Therefore he has suggested that when the remnants of the lingual gingival margin can be located in the edentulous mouth, the cheek position can also deduced by using it as a landmark[8](Fig. 2-46a). As shown in Fig. 2-46b, the average measurement of the buccolingual breadth in the dentate molar region is 10-12 mm. However, after extraction of the teeth, the remnants move outward 3-4 mm from the position in the dentate mouth, so the width of the vestibule should be estimated by deducting this value from the mean buccolingual breadth of dentate patients.

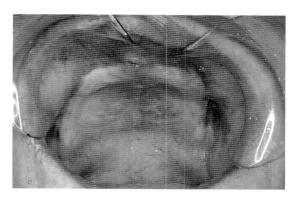

Fig. 2-45 In a severely resorbed ridge, the width of the vestibule is hard to determine.

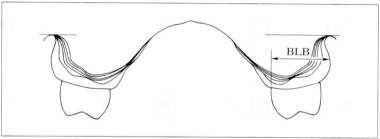

Fig. 2-46a The buccolingual breadth of the dentate alveolar ridge(BLB, horizontal breadth from the lingual gingival margin to the maximal projection of the buccal surface of the alveolar ridge) was remarkably constant for each tooth position(Watt, D.M.).

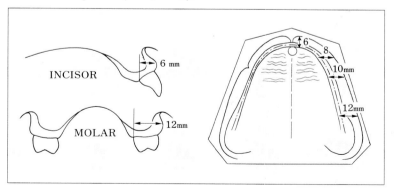

Fig. 2-46b The buccolingual breadth of the alveolar ridge. The remnants of the lingual gingival margin move outwards 3-4 mm after extraction of the teeth, so the width of the vestibule should be estimated by deducting this value from BLB(Watt, D.M.).

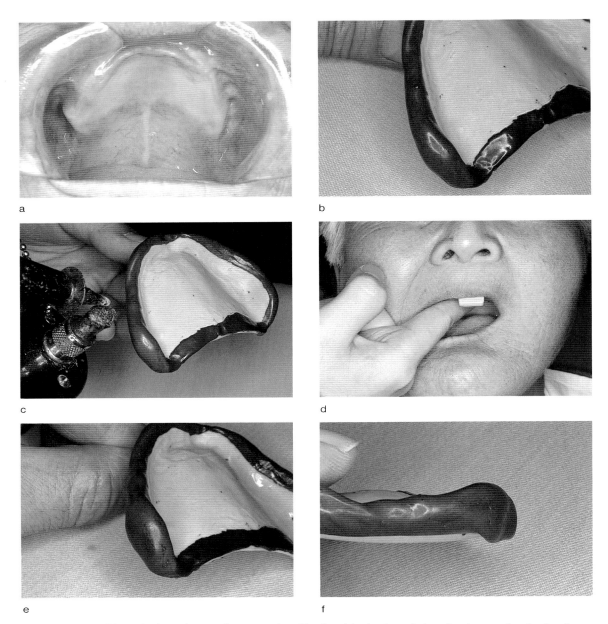

a

b

c

d

e

f

Fig. 2-47a~f   When the buccal space is extremely wide, it might be feared that the denture border has been molded too thickly. The width of the space was recorded just as it was seen(a, b). When this thickness is transferred to the denture border, the coronoid process of the mandible may come into contact with the denture in function. The impression compound should be softened in this area(c), and its width is confirmed by lateral movements of the mandible(d). As contact was present, a shallow concavity was formed on the outer surface of the impression compound(e, f).

As mentioned by Watt, this estimation can not be applied to all cases; however, it can be used as an approximate guide to determine the width of the denture border. In addition, he stated that a slight overestimation of sulcus breadth is preferable to an underestimation. In other words, the additional breadth in the molar region can be accepted because in the dentate patient contact between the cheek and alveolar process may not be present in the molar region. Moreover, the buccinator can act more effectively against a slightly over-molded bulge, leading to an improved buccal seal.

In cases where one is worried that the border may have been molded too thickly, when the thickness is transferred to the denture border, the coronoid process of the mandible may come into contact with the border during function. This should be confirmed by asking the patient to move the jaw laterally after softening the compound on the distobuccal border. If there is any contact, a shallow concavity will be created on the outer surface of the buccal border(Fig. 2-47a〜f).

Posterior border area

The hamular(pterygomaxillary) notch is situated between the maxillary tuberosity and the hamulus of the medial pterygoid plate. It is a favorable landmark for placing the posterior border, which is the most important part for retention of the upper denture(Fig. 2-48). If a mouth mirror or a T-burnisher is slid posteriorly along the crest of the alveolar ridge, its edge will drop into a displaceable depression, the hamular notch-(Fig. 2-49). It can be satisfactorily recorded as there is no muscle or ligament in this notch. If the denture is extended inadequately, the posterior border will be situated on the maxillary tuberosity and a peripheral seal can not be expected from this nonresilient tissue.

The vibrating line(ah-line) runs from one hamular notch to the other across the palate, on which the distal end of the upper denture should be placed. When the patient says "ah" the soft palate rises up and returns to its original position when the patient relaxes. By repeating this movement, the junction of the hard and soft palates(vibrating line) can be recognized as a fold(Fig. 2-50. The hard and soft palates described here mean the clinical ones. See "Clinical junction of the hard and soft palates and its relation to ah-line"). However, the boundary line of movement is not well-defined and is an area rather than a line.

Strictly speaking, the vibrating line is situated slightly posterior to the junction of the hard and soft palates, that is, on the soft palate, thus if the posterior border is placed on this line, the peripheral seal will be established due to the cushion-

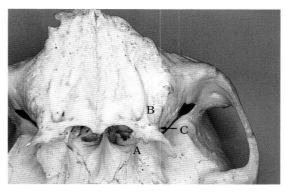

Fig. 2-48 The concavity between the pterygoid hamulus(A) and the maxillary tuberosity(B), the hamular notch(C), is a landmark for placing the posterior border of the upper denture.

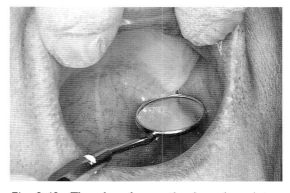

Fig. 2-49 The edge of a mouth mirror drops into a resilient depression, the hamular notch. By using this cushion the peripheral seal can be established.

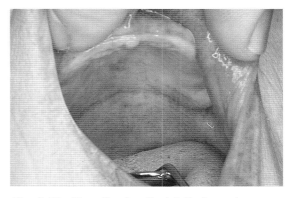

Fig. 2-50 The vibrating line(ah-line) can be recognized as a fold when asking the patient to say"ah" and relax.

The "clinical" junction of the hard and soft palates and its relation to the vibrating line(ah-line)

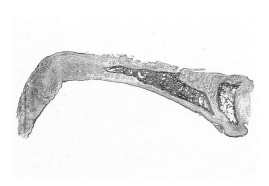

a

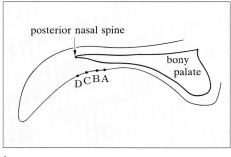

b

Fig. 1a, b Sagittal section through the midline of an edentulous maxilla. a: The hard palate ,which is supported by bone, contains glandular tissue and muscle fibers in the submucosa(by courtesy of Hiroyuki Uchida). b: A＝"clinical" junction of hard and soft palates, B＝ah-line, C＝foveae palatinae, D ＝anatomical junction of hard and soft palates.

In anatomy, the hard and soft palates are distinguished by the existence of bony support. Thus the junction of these two palates is on the distal end of the bony palate. In general, the vibrating line which is used as a posterior guide for the upper denture is considered to coincide with, or be situated somewhat posterior to, this anatomical junction.

The foveae palatinae situated near this junction are also used as a landmark for determining the posterior border of the denture. In anatomy, the foveae palatinae are situated on the distal end of the bony palate or somewhat anterior to it[5,10]. Various reports have described the relation between the foveae palatinae and the vibrating line, perhaps depending upon the various methods of determining the vibrating line. Among the reports, Chen stated that "No foveae palatinae are situated anterior to the vibrating line"[11]. Thus, if the vibrating line is thought as the junction between the movable and immovable portions of the palate, when the patient says "ah", it would be guessed that the vibrating line is located on the anatomical hard palate which is situated anterior to the end of the bony palate.

As shown in Figure 1-a, the hard palate possesses a portion made up of a 4-5 mm thickness of submucosa which contains muscle insertions as well as glandular tissue. Even though the hard palate is supported by bone, it is effected by the levator and tensor muscles of the velum palatini and so it is considered to be movable.

Clinically, from only inspection and palpation, it is difficult to determine whether the palate is supported by bone or not. So, the term, "clinical" hard and soft palates, should be advocated. The hard palate has a firm attachment to the underlying bone, and thus it is hard and immovable on palpation. It is covered by keratinized epithelium, the masticatory mucosa. The soft palate does not lie directly on bone and is soft and movable on palpation. It is covered by non-keratinized epithelium and filled with blood vessels which make it appear red in color. The further it extends posteriorly, the greater the movement is effected by the muscles in the submucosa. The clinical junction of the palates is entirely anterior to the anatomical junction as shown in Figure 1-b. A similar idea is demonstrated in Pendleton's figure in Boucher's textbook, but it does not mention a distinction between the anatomical and clinical junctions and the junction in the textbook seems to be somewhat anterior to the clinical junction mentioned above.

ing effect of the soft palate[9]. Moreover, as mentioned later, if the posterior border is slightly pressed into the mucosa along this line, the valve seal will be improved. This junction can also be located by blowing out through the nose with the nostrils closed in which case the soft palate will expand downwards(Fig. 2-51, nose-blowing method).

Usually the vibrating line passes slightly anterior to the foveae palatinae, thus the posterior border can be determined by using the fovea as a landmark[11](Fig. 2-52).

In the posterior part of the submucosa of the palate, the palatine glands extend anteriorly from the soft palate to the first molar region, taking the shape of a mountain on either side of the midline. The thickness is 4-6 mm in the soft palate and 2-3 mm even in the anterior part on the hard palate[5](Fig. 2-53). Thus there is no need to be anxious regarding how far the posterior border can be extended. If the border is placed only on these palatine glands which possess a cushioning effect, this would be adequate for retention, even if it is placed slightly anteriorly. A little more extension may not lead to much better retention. If it is overdone, the situation will be worse than that of under extension and will lead to a gag reflex and irritation of the movable mucosa. Therefore it is recommended that the posterior border is determined by carefully avoiding the portion moving around the vibrating line whilst saying "ah".

Some clinicians might extend the posterior border posteriorly so as to cover the foveae palatinae by considering the anatomical junction of the two palates, but this concept is not recommended.

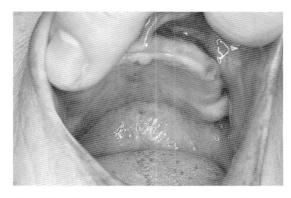

Fig. 2-51 Blowing out through the nose while closing the nostrils causes a downward expansion of the soft palate.

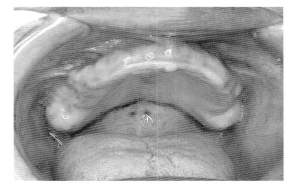

Fig. 2-52 The vibrating line passes slightly anterior to the foveae palatinae.

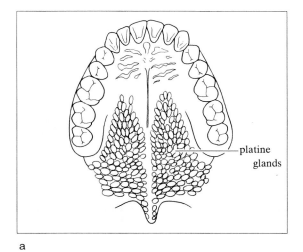

a

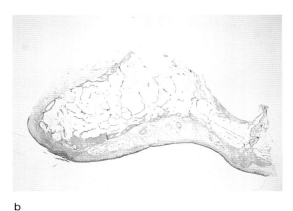

b

Fig. 2-53 a: The palatine glands extend anteriorly from the soft palate to the first molar region taking the shape of a mountain on either side of the midline(From Kamijo, Y.). b: The thickness is 4-6 mm in the soft palate and 2-3 mm in the anterior region(Cross section in the region of the maxillary molars, by courtesy of Hiroyuki Uchida).

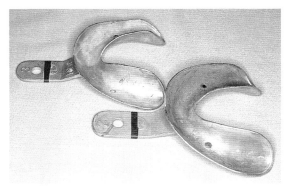

Fig. 2-54 The Britannia metal edentulous tray for modeling compound is also recommended for alginate. This type of tray can be adjusted by cutting and bending, so it is also useful for complicated ridge forms.

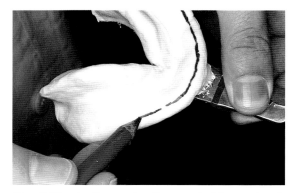

Fig. 2-55 As the maximally extended impression is made using alginate with a stiff or thick consistency, the denture outline is drawn on the impression according to the anatomical landmarks. This will provide important information for the dental technician.

In addition, during border molding, one layer of compound is added on the tissue side of the posterior border of the impression tray and then the tray is seated in the mouth so that additional pressure is applied to this area. In other words, the distal end of the denture will be pressed into the mucosa leading to a better peripheral seal.

3. Preliminary Impression

When making the preliminary impression using a stock tray, a rough but maximally extended impression should be made so as to obtain all the anatomical landmarks. Alginate impression material should be used for the preliminary impression because its manipulation is simple and the setting time is fast, making it a little more pleasant for the patient. In addition, it will not distort the soft tissues because of its soft consistency. However, it is necessary to push away the surrounding tissues to a certain extent in order to capture the anatomical form of the alveolar ridge. For this purpose, the consistency of alginate must be stiff or thick by reducing the amount of water compared with a normal mix.(Fig. 2-55).

When the impression material is to be alginate, an edentulous stock tray for alginate is usually used, but it may be preferable to use the Britannia metal edentulous tray for modeling compound(Nakazawa's tray, Sankin). This type of tray can be adjusted to some degree by cutting and bending even for complicated alveolar ridges. Moreover it is strong and easy to clean(Fig. 2-54). Any deficient tray border should be corrected by adding utility wax.

In the case of a severely resorbed ridge with quite a complicated contour, a rough impression is frequently made with im-

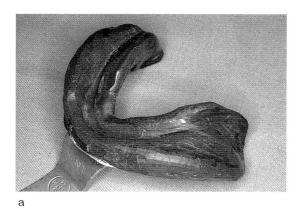
a

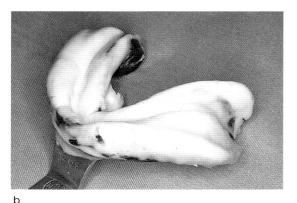
b

Fig. 2-56 a: The inner impression surface of the compound impression is reduced 1-2 mm. b: The alginate impression is made using this compound tray(a).

pression compound and then the inner surface of the impression is reduced to a depth of 1-2mm. This will serve as a preliminary impression tray for alginate(Fig. 2-56a, b).

4. Constructing the individual tray

During the procedure of impression making using a mental image of the completed denture, an appropriate impression will not be made if the tray distorts the tongue, cheeks, lips or floor of the mouth. A stock tray can be used for all kinds of alveolar ridges, but it may not be adaptable in each and every case. Thus a proper impression can not be made with a stock tray (Fig. 2-57).

A preliminary impression is first made with a stock tray and then a preliminary cast is made of artificial stone. A tray which will fit the individual patient is made on this cast. This is called the individual tray. Autopolymerizing acrylic resins are used widely because they can not be distorted by the temperature of the mouth during impression making, and moreover are strong and have good handling characteristics.

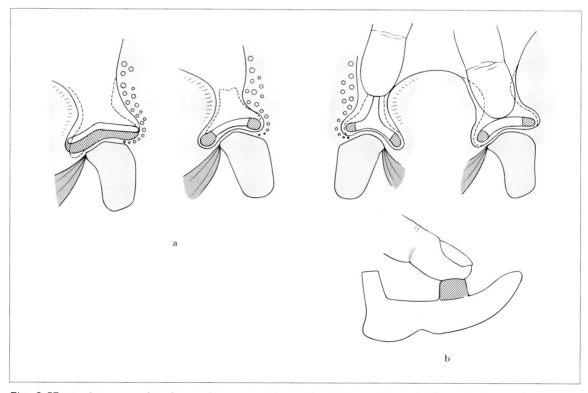

Fig. 2-57 a: An appropriate impression can not be made with a stock tray(left), as it distorts the tongue, cheek, lips or floor of the mouth. An individual tray(right) which mimics the mental image of the completed denture is necessary. b: Finger rests are made bilaterally in the first molar region of the lower individual tray. If the tray is directly held by the fingers, they will distort the tongue and cheeks.

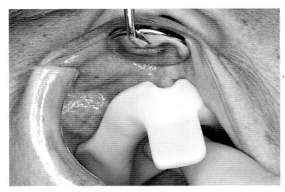

Fig. 2-58 The length of the tray border must be carefully checked inside the mouth prior to border molding.

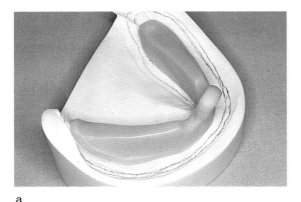

a

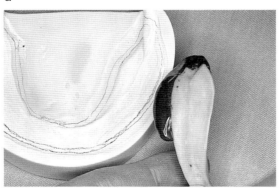

b

Fig. 2-59a, b With an underextended tray, the handling of modeling compound is difficult because of the loss of support due to its increased width.

5. Final impression

When making the preliminary impression, a maximally extended impression is created using alginate with a stiff or thick consistency. Thus, even if the individual tray is made according to the outline of the denture base transferred onto the primary cast(P.135, Fig. 9-37), it tends to be overextended. Therefore, the length of the tray border must be carefully checked in the mouth prior to border molding(Fig. 2-58).

If the length of the tray border is not properly extended, especially if over-extended, border molding is liable to be incorrectly performed. As modeling compound does not flow easily, even if the tray has an overextended area, the modeling compound added on this border will not be completely removed and thus there will be no exposure of tray resin, during border molding. So, this may lead to the mistaken belief that the appropriate border has been apparently recorded. Thus, the method in which modeling compound is added to the tray border on the cast prior to border molding procedure is not recommended. If the tray is underextended, it will be difficult to handle the modeling compound because it can lose support due to its increased width(Fig. 2-59a, b).

Zinc oxide-eugenol paste, being free-flowing, should be used for the final impression. If a rubber base impression material which has a poor flow, such as polysulphide rubber, is used, the border will be extended widely and all the efforts in border molding procedures will have gone with the wind. When a poorly flowing material has to be used, escape channels should be drilled through the palatal part of the upper tray, otherwise it is hard for the impression material to flow out, especially in the maxilla. Excess material will accumulate along the borders. Incidentally, the eugenol contained in the zinc-oxide eugenol impression material is known to be a strong irritant, so it is especially not recommended for use in aged people. Moreover, as the free eugenol is still sticky after setting, the technical procedure is not smooth. A non-eugenol paste having an ideal flow will hopefully be developed soon.

6. Improving the master cast

If the form of the border of the impression is not accurately reproduced on the cast, the whole impression making procedure will come to nothing. Thus, it is essential to correctly box the impression. If boxing is not performed or the height of the land of a boxed cast is too low, the denture border will have to be made by guessing its form(Fig. 2-60). It hardly makes sense to guess the shape of the border because this is important for the peripheral seal. Even in cases where time is limited, beading the border of the impression with utility wax should at least be done prior to pouring the cast(Fig. 2-61).

On the other hand, when boxing is performed, the land of the cast is likely to become higher because generally, too much care is taken to reproduce the impression border accurately on the cast. In other words, it appears that most boxed casts have an extremely deep sulcus. If it is too deep, the following technical procedure, making a baseplate, will be quite difficult. As if the procedure was done with closed eyes, it will not be possible to extend or adapt the baseplate precisely into the sulcus(Fig. 2-62). Naturally, when the land is high, undercuts may occur in a deep sulcus, and thus the land may fracture during fabrication of the baseplate. An inappropriate baseplate will be made and it might lead to an incorrect jaw registration. The portion beyond the most prominent region of the outer surface of the rounded impression border apparently looks like an impression of the tissues, but it is made by excessive flow of impression material during impression making and is not a true record of the mucosal surface. Thus this part of the impression does not need to be restored. This portion will be molded during waxing, becoming the polished surface. Therefore the height of the land should be somewhat higher than the widest region of the sulcus. The edges of the land are slightly tapered and smoothened(Fig. 2-63a, b, 64).

As the cast is made of dental stone, it naturally does not represent the condition of the thickness or resiliency of the mucosa. Therefore an intraoral examination is performed and its condition is written on the cast, and then a plan should be made to cope with the situation. Only after this, does the cast become a "dynamic cast" which takes on life. The measures will vary depending on the impression method used. As the impression technique used in the author's daily practice is almost all nonpressure, measures should be taken to cope with the condition when occlusal forces are applied.

Tinfoil relief is provided accordingly on an area with a thin

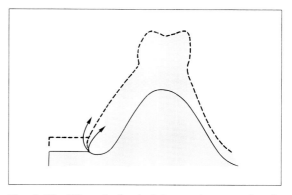

Fig. 2-60   When the land of the cast is over reduced, the form of the denture border must be made by guess work.

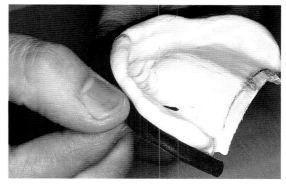

Fig. 2-61   Beading with utility wax should at least be done prior to pouring the cast to reproduce the impression border precisely on the cast.

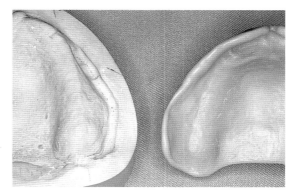

Fig. 2-62   If the land is high, adapting the baseplate into the sulcus will not be possible.

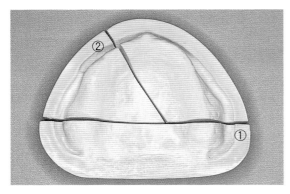

a

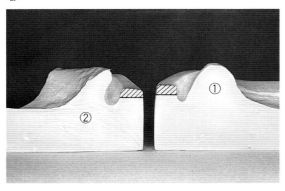

b

Fig. 2-63a, b Cross sections of the cast(Fig. 2-62) at the anterior and posterior regions. The shaded areas are much higher than the widest region(in cross section) of the sulcus and should be eliminated.

covering of mucosa such as a spiny ridge, torus palatinus or torus mandibularis to avoid irritation due to the denture moving towards the tissues(Fig. 2-65). For those areas where the thickness of the mucosa can not be clearly detected by palpation, proper relief should be provided using pressure indicating paste at the time of denture insertion(p. 225).

The post-dam, which is essential for the posterior palatal seal, should be carved along the posterior border region of the upper cast as shown in Fig. 2-66. Additional pressure has already been applied to the posterior border region during impression making. This portion will be projected from the impression surface of the completed denture and it will slightly press into the mucosa leading to an improved palatal seal. So, it may be thought that it is not necessary to improve the palatal seal again by carving the cast. However, the base resin will undergo shrinkage during polymerization and the posterior border may be raised, thereby losing the expected palatal seal. A post-dam should be carved on the cast to compensate for the dimensional changes which occur during polymerization.

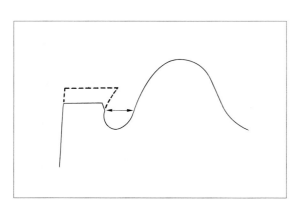

Fig. 2-64 The height of the land should be somewhat higher than the widest region(in cross section) of the sulcus, and a slight bevel is made along the edge of the land.

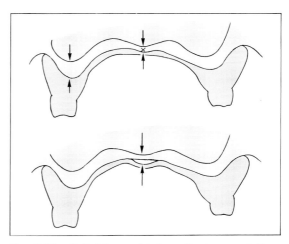

Fig. 2-65 Relief is provided on the torus palatinus covered with thin mucosa to avoid irritation due to the denture moving towards the tissues.

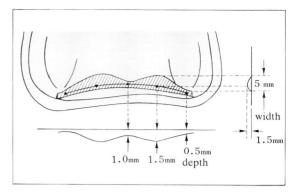

Fig. 2-66 The post-dam is deepest at a point 1/3 of the distance from the posterior edge of the groove and the midpoint between the midline and hamular notches. It becomes gradually shallower anteroposteriorly and laterally.

Chair design for denture patients (1)

During the clinical procedures for denture fabrication, the patient should be in a similar position to that when using dentures owing to their peculiarity. All procedures should be performed with the patient sitting while the operator is standing. However, dental chairs for adults are generally made essentially for the operator to work in the sitting position, and so if the chair is used in a standing position, the operator will not find it very convenient. Moreover, most denture patients are elderly and so this inconvenience might be doubled. As elderly people's posture is different from that of younger adults due to atrophy of the bones and curvature of the spine, the dental chair for adults would be inconvenient for elderly people for the following reasons:

1) If the patient is short, his/her head will rest on the backrest rather than on the headrest. When clinical procedures are performed in a standing position for the operator, both the operator and the patient will have to be in an uncomfortable position (Fig. 1).

2) If the patient's spine is bent, as the height and angle of the headrest can not be freely adjusted, some additional support will be needed.

3) If a rather short patient sits on a knee bend type dental chair with the back of the knee resting against the front edge of the chair, the hips will slide forward and thus the head will slide down the backrest. As a result, the backrest will not support the patient's hips and lower part of the spine, and thus the patient will be seated in an unstable and tiring position. Moreover, as the feet are suspended in the air, the weight of the legs will compress the

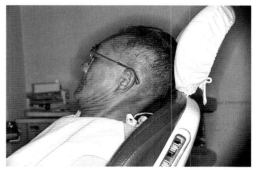

Fig. 1 If the patient is short, the head will rest on the backrest. The headrest can be moved onto the backrest in almost all dental chairs, but is inconvenient for clinical procedures in the standing position.

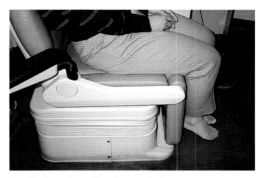

Fig. 2 In a knee bend type chair, when the patient sits with the back of the knee resting against the front edge of the chair, if the femur is short, the hips will slide forward and the backrest will not support the patient's hips and lower part of the spine. The feet will be unsupported and the patient will become tired easily.

Chair design for denture patients (2)

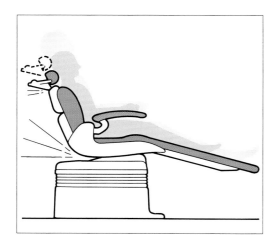

Fig. 3　A chair for denture clinics(Signo S21, Morita Co.). The backrest and headrest can be freely adjusted. The contour type chair can support the weight of the legs.

nerves and vessels of the upper legs and the patient will become tired easily(Fig 2).

To solve these problems, a dental chair for denture fabrication(Signo S21, Morita Co.) has been designed by the author(Fig. 3). The main improvements are as follows:

(1) The backrest can slide up and down, so it may fit any patient height(Fig 4a, b).

(2) The height and angle of the headrest can be freely adjusted, so may be suitable even for patients with a curved spine(Fig 5).

(3) The contour type dental chair, which can support the weight of the legs regardless of their length, is used, so that the patient will not become easily tired even during a long clinical session(Fig 3).

In addition, a micromotor for technical work and a dry vacuum are set in the cart table for improving clinical efficiency.

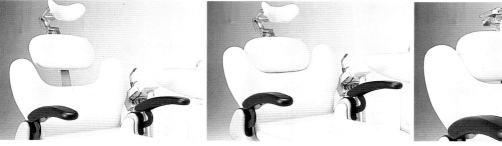

a　　　　　　　　　　　　　　　　　b

Fig. 4　The backrest can slide up and down, so it may fit any patient height.

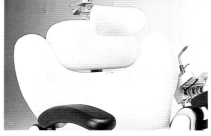

Fig. 5　The height and angle of the headrest can be freely adjusted, so it may be suitable even for patients with a curved spine.

Section 3

Recording the jaw relations

Recording the jaw relations

Recording the jaw relations and impression making are two important steps for the success of complete dentures. But if one asks the question "Which is more important?", recording the jaw relations must be considered to be more important. Everyone may have experienced that an impression was perfect, such that it was difficult to remove the denture from the ridge when the upper and lower dentures were inserted separately, but when the jaw relations were incorrect, the dentures became gradually loose on repeated occlusion and finally were dislodged. On the contrary, even if the impression is a little deficient and thus the retention of the denture becomes poor, when the jaw relations are corrected, the dentures can be used for a while due to the retention which can be reasonably improved.

If the jaw relations are incorrect, the dentures will move to occlude with each other and thus be dislodged from the ridges during occlusion. By the way, if the mucosa of the alveolar ridge is resilient, the denture will bounce away upon each application and release of the occlusal forces. Fortunately, recovery of the displaced mucosa takes place slowly due to its viscoelasticity. So, if the jaw relations are correct and the denture is repeatedly pushed into the mucosa during occlusion, the denture will seat into the mucosa. Therefore, retention of the denture base will be sustained.

However, "jaw relations" are somewhat tricky. Occasionally, it appears that nothing is wrong at the try-in stage, but when the dentures are inserted, one is surprised to find that the occlusion is poor. The recording method which is widely performed using the denture base and occlusion rim requires skill and thus is difficult to perform correctly. The method in which the gothic arch tracer is used is simple and appropriate and thus should be recommended for beginners although here, a further step will be included in its construction.

The term "bite taking" is generally used for recording the

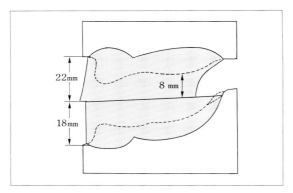

Fig. 3-1   The average height of the occlusion rims-(Jamieson, C.H.[12]). Upper rim: 22 mm high from the labial sulcus of the cast, 8 mm above the crest of the ridge in the second molar region. Lower rim: 18 mm from the labial sulcus, 1/2 the height of the retromolar pad in the posterior region.

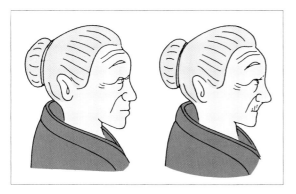

Fig. 3-2   Many upper occlusion rims with inadequate labial fullness are found. If the upper lip is not adequately supported, it will mislead the determination of the occlusal vertical dimension. If the support of the upper lip is insufficient, even with the same height of occlusion rim, the occlusal vertical dimension will appear smaller(right).

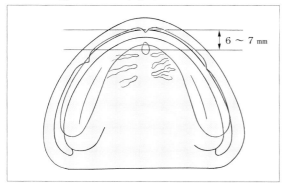

Fig. 3-3   An average degree of labial fullness must be given by referring to the incisive papilla. The labial surface of the occlusion rim should be 6-7 mm anterior to the middle of the incisive papilla.

jaw relations, however the edentulous jaw bears no teeth to bite and therefore the sense of biting becomes obscure. It is appropriate to say "recording the jaw relations". Recording the relations between the upper and lower jaws requires the dentist and patient to seek one point in the 3 dimensional movements of the lower jaw. It can be obtained by recording the vertical and horizontal relationships of the lower jaw to the upper jaw. It is performed clinically in such a way that initially the occlusal vertical dimension is determined and then the anteroposterior and lateral relations of the lower jaw are recorded at the determined occlusal vertical dimension.

1. Constructing the baseplates and occlusion rims

The relationships of the lower jaw with the upper jaw can not be directly recorded in edentulous cases. Baseplates and occlusion rims are needed for recording the jaw relations. They must be strong enough to bear the occlusal force and made of materials which will not be deformed by the temperature of the mouth. Considering the handling properties, generally the baseplates which cover the alveolar ridges are made of shellac baseplate material or autopolymerizing resins and the occlusion rims are made of modelling wax.

When making bases and rims, average dimensions are given to the occlusion rims prior to trying them in the patient's mouth. The height varies in each case because it corresponds to the crown length of the missing teeth plus the amount of bone resorption after the teeth are lost. However, if average dimensions are given to the occlusion rims, correction during the recording of jaw relations will be minimized and thus the chairtime will be shortened(Fig. 3-1). The degree of labial fullness of the occlusion rim, especially in the upper lip region, will directly influence the determination of the occlusal vertical dimension. When the labial support is inadequate, the appearance will be spoiled, and it will mislead the determination of the occlusal vertical dimension(Fig. 3-2). An average degree of labial fullness must be given by using the incisive papilla as a landmark(Fig. 3-3).

2. Determining the occlusal plane

The tentative occlusal plane, which represents the level at which the artificial teeth will be set, is determined by referring to the relationships between the natural teeth and the skull and face in the dentition and thence by imagining the occlusal plane of the completed denture. Many reports have described reference lines used for determining the occlusal plane.

However, Camper's plane is used most frequently in clinical practice. This plane is established by a line(Camper's line, ala-tragus line) passing from the lowest point of the ala of the nose to the center of the tragus of the ear(The posterior reference point varies with researchers; some prefer the superior or inferior margin of the tragus, while others prefer the superior or inferior border of the external auditory meatus[13,14]). In clinical practice, an upper baseplate with an occlusion rim is inserted into the mouth and anteriorly, the occlusion rim is adjusted to the level of the lower border of the upper lip and then trimmed until the occlusal plane is parallel to the interpupillary line when viewed from the front and also parallel to Camper's line when viewed from the side. However, when the posterior teeth are set on this occlusion rim adjusted parallel to Camper's line, the posterior occlusal plane may not coincide with the ideal set up of the teeth and so it has to be frequently modified on the articulator. Recently, in many papers it has been reported that Camper's line is not parallel to the occlusal plane and is being questioned as to whether it is an accurate guide for orientating the occlusal plane[14,15]. It has also been found to diverge posteriorly by the author[16]. This tentative occlusal plane can provide a rough guide for the vertical position of the upper anterior teeth and be effective in leveling the height of the right and left sides of the occlusal plane, but it is not appropriate for the arrangement of the posterior teeth without carrying out any modifications. Therefore, clinically, oral anatomical landmarks should also be used to reproduce the occlusal plane of the natural teeth. Moreover, some adjustments are made after mounting on the articulator according to the vertical relation of the upper and lower alveolar ridges(Fig. 3-4a~c).

The reason why it is inconvenient in a case where the occlusal plane inclines towards the alveolar ridge is that when it is higher in the molar region and tips anteriorly(Fig. 3-5), the upper denture tends to move anteriorly and the lower denture posteriorly due to the occlusal force. In other words, a shunting effect occurs, leading to a loss of denture stability. If the occlusal plane is higher in the anterior region and is tipping posteriorly, the shunting effect will be the opposite. When the teeth are set depending only on the tentative occlusal plane parallel to Camper's line, the occlusal plane of the denture may easily incline as mentioned above.

Mistakes will not be made when leveling the height of the right and left sides of the occlusion rims, if the interpupillary line, tragi or earlobes are used as references. But if there is a discrepancy in their heights, the balance of the denture will be affected and a lateral shunting effect will occur.

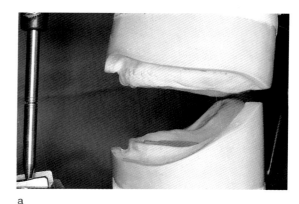

a

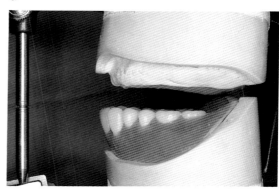

b

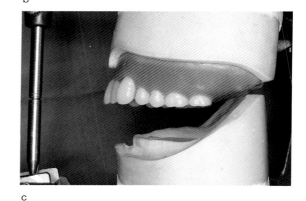

c

Fig. 3-4a ~ c The tentative occlusal plane is adjusted even after mounting on the articulator, to reproduce the occlusal plane of the natural teeth by referring to anatomical landmarks. Ideally, if it is parallel to the upper and lower alveolar ridges, the denture will gain optimum stability.

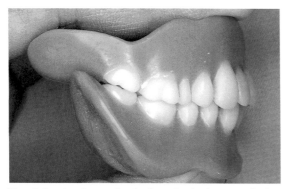

Fig. 3-5 As the occlusal plane is tipping anteriorly, due to occlusal forces, the upper denture moves anteriorly and the lower denture moves posteriorly.

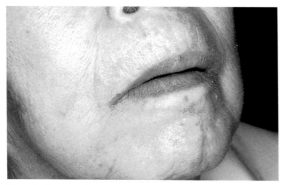

Fig. 3-6 As the occlusal vertical dimension is too great, the face looks distorted and the lips are incompetent.

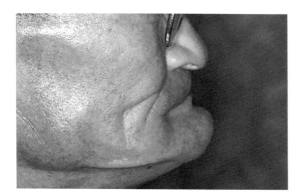

Fig. 3-7 As the occlusal vertical dimension is too small, the vermilion border appears thin and wrinkles occur around the lips. The chin is apparently protruded.

Of course, these shunting effects will also occur during the recording of the jaw relations and so the upper and lower occlusion rims may slip during contact leading to a mistake. The inclination of the occlusion rims should be corrected as much as possible prior to recording the centric occlusal position.

3. Determining the occlusal vertical dimension

In edentulous cases, as there are no teeth, it is almost impossible to reproduce the occlusal vertical dimension of the dentate condition. Generally in practice, dentists easily find a so-called "proper occlusal vertical dimension" using various techniques. The occlusal vertical dimension provided for an edentulous patient varies with each practitioner and also its range is considerably wide. However, major problems are unlikely to occur and therefore every denture can be successful. Of course, there must be an appropriate occlusal vertical dimension for each patient, but the permissible range for the vertical relation is wider than the horizontal relation. Thus the proper, clinically acceptable, occlusal vertical dimension is better referred to as a "zone".

It is sufficient to determine the occlusal vertical dimension in the zone, so the author easily records it without considering any minor matters, by referring to the morphological harmony of the face, namely the appearance. Functional methods determining the occlusal vertical dimension by using the rest position of the mandible, biting force, swallowing movement or phonetics are effective, but they are affected by the skill, mental tension and posture of the patient and also by the quality and stability of the occlusion rims. In other words, these methods are complicated and easily lead to errors. The method for determining the occlusal vertical dimension from the aspect of appearance needs a little skill, but if the operator becomes accustomed to it, the occlusal vertical dimension will be determined quickly without bothering the patient or being affected by various situations. If the appearance is in harmony, the occlusal vertical dimension will be close to that in the dentate condition.

Dentists have been observing the human face with much more attention than other people and so they should be especially skillful in grasping the appearance of the area around the mouth. Therefore, visual assessment ought to be reliable in determining the occlusal vertical dimension.

The author would like to briefly describe this method for the beginner. If the occlusal vertical dimension is too great, the lower third of the face will look longer and the lips will be incompetent(Fig. 3-6). If the occlusal vertical dimension is too small, the lips will be strongly sealed and the lip line will be lengthened. The vermilion border will become thin and wrinkles will occur on the lips. The chin will be apparently too far forward(Fig. 3-7). As the occlusal vertical dimension is thought of as a zone, it will be adequate if recorded between the above two situations. If the patient has a picture taken when the teeth were present, the appearance of the lower facial region can be assessed using the photograph. However, as mentioned previously, this method is prone to error when the labial fullness of the upper occlusion rim is inappropriate and therefore attention is required so as to gain the correct fullness.

In this way, the occlusal vertical dimension is determined by allowing the face to have the most appropriate morphological height using occlusion rims. Afterwards the vertical dimension is reduced a little. From the author's experience, it seems that the prognosis is not good when the occlusal vertical dimension in the dentate condition is given to the patient. For a case with severe bone resorption, sometimes the vertical dimension is reduced much more with the aim of reducing the occlusal force. Normally the occlusal vertical dimension should be reduced 2-3 mm from the appropriate morphological height.

The prediction formula for the vertical dimension and the OVD Indicator (1)

As mentioned above, the occlusal vertical dimension is determined by the morphological harmony of the face, the appearance. However, there should be some concern as to whether the optimum vertical dimension is given precisely or not. Fortunately, as the permissible range of the vertical dimension is rather wide, success is possible.

However, for beginners, although the range is wide, it seems difficult to grasp even this range accurately. For determining the occlusal vertical dimension, a device like a Gothic arch tracer for determining the horizontal relation, which can decide the vertical dimension objectively and easily, has not yet been developed. The author has devised a prediction formula and designed the OVD Indicator(Onuki Dental Co.) for applying the formula clinically[17,18].

1) The prediction formula for the occlusal vertical dimension

The prediction formula was devised from the multiple regression analysis of the measurements on the face concerning the vertical dimension and additional information obtained from facial form and the palm of

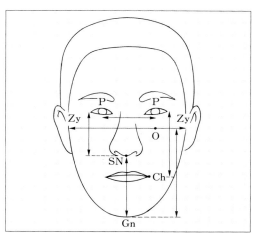

Fig. 1-a   The measuring points used for prediction. P(pupil point), the center of the pupil of the eye; Zy(zygomatic point), the most lateral point of the surface of the zygomatic process(the intersection point of the tragus and the center line of the index finger which is put into the external auditory meatus is used for convenience); SN(subnasion), the inferior border of the center of the nose; Ch(cheilion), the left corner of the mouth; Gn(gnathion), the inferior border of the chin.

The prediction formula for the vertical dimension and the OVD Indicator (2)

SN-Gn(the distance from SN to Gn) $= 3.95 + 1.16 \times$ (gender) $+ 1.45 \times$ (profile) $+ 0.11 \times$ (the length of the palm) $+ 0.91 \times$ (p-Ch) $+ 0.10 \times$ (p-p) $+ 0.10 \times$ (Zy-Zy) $- 0.93 \times$ (p-SN) [unit mm]

gender male 1, female 0; profile convex 1, straight 2, concave 3.

Fig. 1-b   Prediction formula

the hand(Fig. 1a, b).

This prediction formula possesses a multiple coefficient of determination $R^2 = 0.634$. This formula may be effective in predicting the vertical dimension. In the method using this formula, many measuring points are used, so the procedure is rather complicated, but even if some measuring points are somewhat mistaken, its affect on the calculated value will be minimal.

Simplified method

SN-Gn $= 16.0 + 0.65 \times$ (p-Ch) [unit mm]

Zy-Gn $= 24.6 +$ (p-Ch) [unit mm]

The above two formulas can be used as rough guides for determining the vertical dimension when there is insufficient time to measure all the points.

2) OVD Indicator

Procedure

(1) Position the head so that the Frankfort horizontal

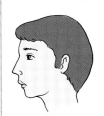 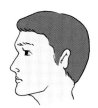 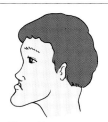

The upper lip region protrudes.

The forehead, the base of the nose and the chin are in line.

The chin protrudes and the upper lip region retrudes.

Fig. 2   The profile of the face. convex 1, straight 2, concave 3.

plane is parallel to the floor. Place the indicator on the face so that the nose comes through the center triangle and then rest the subnasion on the center of the triangle's base. Hold the plate perpendicularly and ask the patient to look straight ahead.

(2) Classify the profile of the face as convex, straight or concave(Fig. 2).

(3) Measure the distance from the center of the pupil to the corner of the mouth(p-Ch) and the distance from the center of the pupil to the inferior border of the nose(p-SN)(Fig. 3).

(4) Rotate the plate and fit the V-shaped notch to the bridge of the nose. Measure the distance between the pupils(p-p) and the distance between the zygomatic points(Zy-Zy)(Fig. 4, 5).

(5) Measure the length of the left palm(Fig. 6).

(6) Enter all the measured values, and the index values of the profile of the face and gender into the formula and then calculate the predicted distance

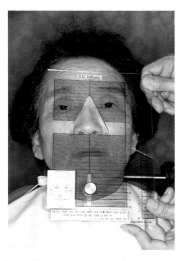

Fig. 3   Place SN on the center of the triangle's base and measure the distances, p-Ch and p-SN.

The prediction formula for the vertical dimension and the OVD Indicator (3)

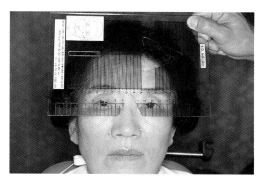

Fig. 4 Rotate the plate and place the V-shaped notch over the bridge of the nose. Measure the distance, p-p.

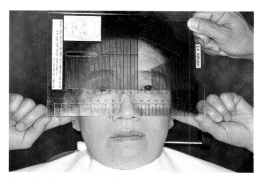

Fig. 5 Put the index fingers into both external auditory meatuses. The intersection point of the tragus and the center of the finger is called the zygomatic point, Zy and measure the distance, Zy-Zy.

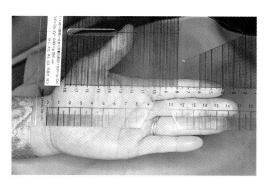

Fig. 6 Measure the length of the left palm.

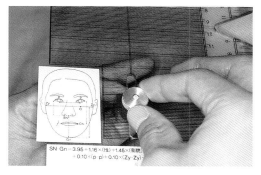

Fig. 7 Enter all measured values, and the index values of the profile and gender into the formula. Calculate to predict the distance, SN-Gn and transfer the predicted value to the scale.

from the inferior border of the nose to the inferior border of the chin(SN-Gn). Insert the occlusion rims and replace the indicator on the face. Slide the red indicator bar up to the position beneath the gnathion and read the scale. Correct the occlusion rim by referring to the calculated dimension(Fig. 7, 8).

Characteristics
(1) Measuring points can be read precisely by overlapping the lines with each other, which are drawn on both sides of the measuring plate.
(2) When using ordinary measuring devices, the measured distance may vary with differences in the inclination of the device, so the reference distance can not be applied precisely for the occlusal vertical dimension. In the OVD Indicator, all measured distances can be indicated on the same plane.
(3) The measuring points and the formula are shown on the indicator.
(4) The indicator can be applied to all the morphological determination methods such as Willis' method and Bruno's method.

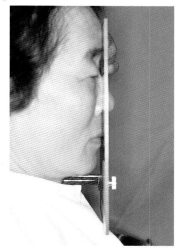

Fig. 8 Insert the occlusion rims into the mouth and place the indicator on the face. Slide the red bar up to the position beneath the gnathion and read the scale. Correct the occlusion rim by referring to the predicted value.

This is performed simultaneously when recording the centric occlusal position. By the way, in a patient wearing a denture with an extremely reduced occlusal vertical dimension for a long time, the new denture may fail if the occlusal vertical dimension is increased too much. The occlusal vertical dimension should be gradually increased by repeatedly fabricating the dentures. Self-curing acrylic resin is also used to gradually build up the posterior occlusal surfaces of the existing denture, and then after the patient has become accustomed to the desired height, a new denture should be made at this height.

4. Recording the centric occlusal position

The mandibular position must be recorded so that maximum occlusal contact can be made to coincide with it. As the vertical relation has already been established, the horizontal relation is determined using the same occlusion rims. The recording of the jaw relations is then complete. The upper and lower casts are mounted on an articulator using the records.

The horizontal relation does not have a permissible range unlike the vertical relation and thus must be precisely recorded. When carried out accurately, the dentures will have complete intercuspation in the centric occlusal position. Therefore the denture is pushed into the mucosa repeatedly during occlusion, improving its retention. However, if the recording is incorrect, the occlusal force will create a dislodging force to the denture. In order to obtain the record more precisely, the gothic arch tracing method, together with the tapping point record, is recommended.

Whether complete dentures should be constructed with the occlusion harmonious with centric relation(the most retruded position) or a little anteriorly to it, the centric occlusal position(the centric occlusion), has been debated for a long time. The author wants to briefly mention some issues. The situation where the centric occlusal position of the dentate person does not coincide with centric relation could be considered a minor malocclusion. By nature, the teeth should occlude in the most retruded position. After all the teeth are lost, the most retruded position of the jaw is the only position which can be accurately obtained and reproduced. For these reasons, centric relation is assumed to be the optimum occlusal position for edentulous patients.[9] Others advocate that dentures should occlude in the centric occlusal position according to the following reasons[19]. The most retruded position of the jaw, centric relation, is just a border position. In other words, it is a forced position. Usually the joint movements of the body are performed far inside of the border movements except when consciously moved. A functional movement is never performed at the border position. During the movements of mastication, the masticatory stroke ends in the centric occlusal position, not in centric relation[20]. It is impossible to force the functional movements to end in centric relation.

So far a clear conclusion of the discussion has not been reached, but the author agrees with the latter concept of the centric occlusal position. In daily complete denture practice, as the denture may settle or displace due to the compressibility of the alveolar ridge, it is difficult to ascertain which is better. In other words, a serious problem will not occur even if the dentures occlude in either position. It is only important that the clinician should have an idea in which position the dentures ought to occlude.

It is necessary to know how to record the centric occlusal position clinically, which is thought to be the end-point of a functional movement. Repeatedly performed unconsious opening and closing movements of the jaw are called the habitual opening and closing movements. They are thought to end in the centric occlusal position[20,21](Fig. 3-8). By tapping the occlusion rims together, the centric occlusal position can be

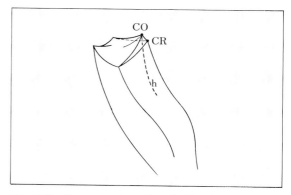

Fig. 3-8 The end-point of the habitual opening and closing movement is thought to coincide with the centric occlusal position. It can be found from repeated movements on the habitual opening and closing movement path, namely tapping.

Determining the mandibular position by the operator's guidance and habitual chewing

In an edentulous patient with a habitual chewing side, when the mandible is guided by the operator during recording of the horizontal jaw relations, the mandibular position may be recorded on the habitual chewing side.

Figure 1 shows the positions recorded by the operator's guidance(the operator's clinical experience is just three years) and the Gothic arch tracings of 12 edentulous patients with a definite habitual chewing side. After performing the Gothic arch tracings, the guided mandibular positions were then transferred onto the tracing plates. In 9 out of 12 cases, the mandibular positions were recorded on the habitual chewing side. Therefore it is suggested that the operator's guidance method is easily influenced by habitual chewing[22].

If the clinician is familiar with the guidance method, no problem will occur. However, the beginner is recommended to use the Gothic arch tracer. The tapping points and the Gothic arch tracings should be recorded and then the appropriate tapping point can be objectively determined by referring to the Gothic arch tracings.

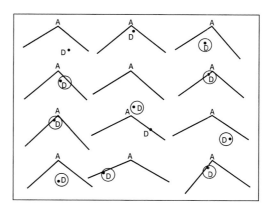

Fig. 1 The gothic arch tracings and the mandibular positions recorded by the operator's guidance in patients with a definite habitual chewing side(Lin, C.). A, the apex of the Gothic arch tracings; D, the mandibular position obtained by the operator's guidance(Ⓓ, the mandibular position obtained on the habitual chewing side).

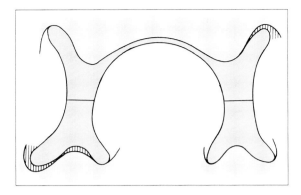

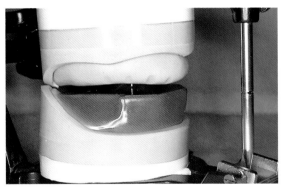

a

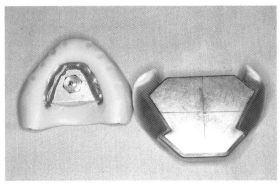

b

Fig. 3-10a, b   As the Gothic arch tracer is supported at the central-bearing point the force will be evenly transmitted to the alveolar ridges through the bases. In order to avoid displacement of the bases, the stylus must not be attached off-center of the alveolar ridge.

found from the repeated movements on the habitual opening and closing movement path. Centric occlusal position can almost certainly be reproduced, even in edentulous cases, if correct techniques are used.

5. Gothic arch tracing method

The method of recording the jaw relationships using baseplates and occlusion rims, as mentioned above, is widely carried out in clinical practice. However, as many dentures with an unstable occlusion are seen, it is thought that minor errors tend to occur easily using this technique. There are various reasons to explain this. If the clinician is not accustomed to the procedure of softening the wax, it will be difficult to soften the rims evenly. Without uniformly softened rims, an exact record can not be expected. When the baseplates poorly fit the alveolar ridges, they are displaced by sliding over the occlusal plane during recording and thus the jaw registration is carried out with displaced rims. In addition, as the mucosa of the alveolar ridge is compressible, some portions of the baseplate settles into the mucosa slightly and another portion is raised up, but this depends on the case. In a case with severe ridge resorption, the baseplate will be easily displaced. In a patient with a loose temporomandibular joint or wearing an existing denture with a malocclusion for a long time, the eccentric relation might be easily recorded by a little undue pressure.

After the registration, some dentists try to examine the displacement of the baseplates by separating the upper and lower occlusion rims with a spatula. This is useful for detecting a huge displacement. However, when the displacement is small, the record looks apparently correct even for the experienced clinician, who may fail to find it. As a result, a lot of time will be needed for adjusting the occlusion of the completed denture. It should be called the "apparent jaw registration"(Fig. 3-9).

In any case, it requires great skill for the horizontal and vertical jaw relations to be recorded simultaneously just by using the baseplates to establish an exact jaw relationship. The chairtime will also be prolonged, and thus the physical fatigue of the patient will increase. To solve these problems, the author divides the procedure into two stages. The gothic arch tracer is used for recording the horizontal jaw relation. The patient must come to the clinic once more, but as the final decision can be left to the use of the gothic arch tracer, the procedure for recording the vertical relation using baseplates can be performed stress-free and moreover the total chairtime for the recording jaw relations is shortened.

1) Mounting the Gothic arch tracer

Using the tentative jaw relation record, obtained with the baseplates and occlusion rims, the upper and lower casts are temporarily mounted on the articulator. The record bases are made on the casts and then the gothic arch tracer is mounted on the bases. As the gothic arch tracer is supported at one point, the central-bearing point, the force will be evenly transmitted to the alveolar ridges through the bases and unlike in the baseplate technique, displacement of the baseplates will not occur any more. However, if the needle point tracer is attached off center of the alveolar ridge, the record bases will tend to raise up. In addition, as the level and orientation of the tracing plate may be culprits in creating errors, care should be taken during the mounting of the gothic arch tracer(Fig. 3-10a, b).

2) Tracing the Gothic arch and the tapping point

When a tracing is made in the dentition, two Gothic arch tracings are obtained; the apex of one tracing indicates the centric relation and the other indicates the centric occlusal position[23,24]. Therefore, it is possible in edentulous cases to obtain either tracing depending on the guiding techniques. Sometimes tracings may be obtained with a dull or rounded apex by improper posterior movement of the mandible or movement of the recording bases on their basal seats. When the tracing is made by instructing the patient to retrude the mandible consciously, as this action is in the horizontal plane, the patient can pull the mandible posteriorly more easily than in three-dimensional movements. Thus it is quite possible to obtain the centric relation. If the tracing is made unconsciously, the apex may coincide with the centric occlusal position. However this is uncertain. As the tracing plate limits the vertical portion of the three-dimensional movements of the lower jaw, the movement is confined only to the horizontal plane, which is not representative of the actual movements of the mandible. Therefore the end-point of the functional movements of the mandible can not be grasped exactly.

The patient should be instructed to lightly perform opening and closing movements in the posterior region after the Gothic arch tracer assembly is inserted. When the marked points concentrate on one point on the tracing plate, this point indicates the centric occlusal position. The three-dimensional movements of the lower jaw are reproduced by light tapping on the habitual closing movement path and the end-point of the movement, centric occlusal position, is recorded

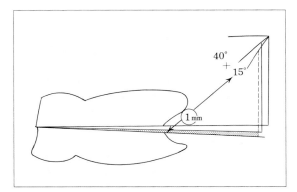

Fig. 3-11   When recording the protrusive occlusion by an intraoral protrusive record, 0.5 mm compression of the mucosa in both upper and lower jaws causes a 1 mm change in the vertical dimension of the register in the posterior region, resulting in a 15 degree error in the sagittal condylar guidance angle adjustment (Watt, D.M. & MacGregor, A.R.).

in the horizontal plane. Initially these points are scattered, but as the patient becomes accustomed to this procedure, the muscles become relaxed and these points gradually concentrate towards one point. The situation when the scattered points concentrate on one point is a signal for establishing the recording of the centric occlusal position.

In some cases, even if the tapping points concentrate on one point, this will not indicate the centric occlusal position. This is a case of "habitual eccentric occlusion". When the patient has worn inappropriate dentures for a long time, the occlusion is habitually out of the centric occlusal position due to the functional adaptation of the body in which one masticates in a position comfortable to him/herself. The Gothic arch tracing should be made and the apex is compared with the tapping point to find their relation. If two points are within 1-2 mm, no problem will occur. But if the two points are far apart, it will be necessary to correct it gradually using treatment dentures.

6. Articulators and mounting casts

As a prosthesis is made indirectly on an articulator, needless to say, the articulator is expected to imitate the mandibular movements of the patient as much as possible. Nowadays, some articulators which can almost completely replicate the mandibular movements have been developed. However, when the peculiarity of the prosthesis for an edentulous case is considered, the mean value articulator is acceptable for complete denture construction and is recommended.

In order to precisely reproduce the mandibular movements using an adjustable articulator, it is necessary to have accurate registration procedures and fine adjustment of the articulator. However, in an edentulous case, although the recording plates are retentive, they are not firmly fixed to the residual ridges but only placed on them. Thus they might easily move during the recording procedures and also be affected by the compressibility of the oral mucosa, leading to an error in the registration procedure. For example, when registering the protrusive occlusion with an intraoral protrusive record, 0.5 mm compression in both upper and lower jaws produces a 1.0 mm change in the vertical dimension of the register in the molar region. As a result, a 15 degree error will occur in the sagittal condylar guidance angle adjustment(Fig. 3-11). Similar errors can not be avoided when locating the hinge axis. Moreover, errors might occur in adjusting the articulator depending on the materials used for the interocclusal records[8].

In complete denture fabrication, it makes no sense using an

articulator with complicated condylar elements, when pantographic records of the mandibular movements are used. It will only increase the work with very little benefit. On the other hand, the condylar guidance of a mean value articulator can not be adjusted for each patient, but as it is designed to reproduce average mandibular movements, it will accommodate most patients without causing any major clinical errors. Because of its simplicity, it is a pleasure to handle.

In a case with favorable residual ridges, the record plates are more stable and thus a semi-adjustable articulator may be used. Certainly the semi-adjustable articulator is appropriate to study the jaw movements and it might be just suited to surprise the patient. But preferably, the registration of the condylar path angle and the articulator adjustment should be performed using the completed dentures with artificial teeth, whose fit is improved.

Split-cast method

In order to accurately replace the cast on the articulator after processing and to correct any changes in occlusion which may occur during processing, the split-cast method should be used. Usually, occlusal equilibration is done subsequently. Grooves or notches are made in the base of the cast for indexing.

Section 4

Arranging the artificial teeth

Arranging the artificial teeth

Masticatory movements in the dentate state are controlled by the mutual cooperation of the teeth, temporomandibular joints and muscles which are entirely regulated by the central nervous system. If the teeth are lost, naturally, the masticatory system will be disrupted. However, even in the complete absence of teeth the regulatory system of muscle activity of the masticatory movements continues as before. Thus if only the teeth are replaced, in other words, if the occlusion is restored using artificial teeth, the masticatory movement mechanism of the dentate state will resume and mastication will recover after a short time, although it will temporarily be somewhat confused at first. Now, where and how should the artificial teeth be set ? This is the point of artificial tooth arrangement.

Successful dentures require that the artificial teeth be placed in the position occupied by the natural teeth.

However, regarding the artificial tooth arrangement, generally the relationship of the teeth to the ridge is considered, and the lever system which is created between the teeth and ridge seems to be the only thing that dentists pay attention to. Thus it is suggested that optimum denture stability is obtained when the artificial teeth are placed on, or lingual to, the residual ridge(Fig. 4-1). However, if this principle is strictly adhered to, in accordance with the direction of the alveolar bone resorption, inevitably the teeth will be placed more lingual to the position occupied by the natural teeth and thus the tongue space will be encroached upon. In addition, the support for the lips and cheeks will be inadequate. As a result, the tongue will push the denture and thus the denture becomes unstable, nullifying the original objectives. The phonetics and esthetics will also be severely affected.

The lever system is only an armchair theory based on mechanical principles. The dentures will be used in the mouth and thus attention must be paid to the environment where the dentures function and care must be taken to maintain har-

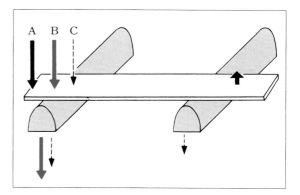

Fig. 4-1 If the artificial teeth are arranged on A, the occlusal load placed on A will serve as the tilting force with a fulcrum on the ridge crest. If arranged on B or C, the occlusal load will serve to place the denture in position leading to stability of the denture.

Problems of the interalveolar ridge line theory(1)

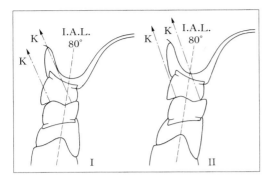

Fig. 1   If the artificial teeth are arranged buccally to the interalveolar ridge line as seen in I, the denture will be dislodged because the tilting force(K) will exert far outside the buccal border of the denture. To avoid this, the teeth are arranged as near as possible to the interalveolar ridge line as in II(Gysi, A.).

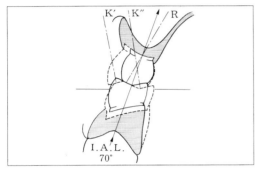

Fig. 2   When the interalveolar ridge line is severely inclined inward, the tilting force(K) will be more predominant than the retentive force(R)(dotted line) and the denture will be dislodged. In the case where the interalveolar ridge line is inclined at less than 80 degrees to the occlusal plane, a cross-bite arrangement of the teeth should be set up(Gysi, A.).

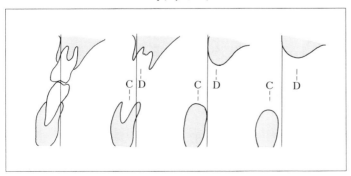

Fig. 3   After the upper posterior teeth are lost, alveolar bone resorption occurs upward and inward and thus the alveolar ridge becomes progressively smaller inward. In the lower jaw, according to resorption, the ridge seems to move somewhat buccally(From Boucher's prosthodontic treatment for edentulous patients).

As is generally known, the line which connects the crests of the upper and lower alveolar ridges is called the interalveolar ridge line. "The interalveolar ridge line theory" is defined as arranging the posterior artificial teeth on or lingually to the interalveolar ridge line to maintain the mechanical balance of the dentures. In other words, when such an arrangement is set up, a unilaterally balanced occlusion is considered to be obtained when food is chewed on one side(Fig. 1).

In the case of severe alveolar ridge resorption, the upper arch is extremely reduced and the interalveolar ridge line is inclined inward. Thus, even if the teeth are arranged on this line, the denture will be dislodged because the tilting forces on the maxillary buccal facets become more active. Therefore, in a case where the interalveolar ridge line is inclined at less than 80 degrees to the occlusal plane, the teeth are arranged in a cross-bite configuration[25](Fig. 2).

As shown in Figure 3, the inclination of the upper posterior teeth is downward and outward, thus alveolar bone resorption occurs upward and inward after the teeth are lost. In addition, as the buccal alveolar bone is thinner than that on the lingual side, faster and greater buccal resorption occurs. As a result, the upper alveolar ridge becomes progressively smaller moving inwards. On the other hand, in the mandible, as the lingual plate of alveolar bone resorbs after extraction, the ridge seems to move somewhat buccally as the resorption progresses.[9] Therefore in most cases with severe alveolar ridge resorption, the angle between the interalveolar ridge line and the occlusal plane is less than 80 degrees. So a cross-bite arrangement must be set up when the resorption has progres-

Problems of the interalveolar ridge line theory (2)

sed. In fact, the cross-bite arrangement is often seen in severe alveolar ridge resorption cases and it is felt that many clinicians try to arrange the teeth on a mechanical basis.

The opinion of arranging the teeth on the crest of the residual ridge based on the mechanical theory is strongly supported by many dentists like an established theory or an unquestioning belief as a requirement for denture stability. The interalveolar ridge line theory is representative of the mechanical theories. As this theory is based on the simple lever system, it is easy to understand and as such is very persuasive. However, no consideration is given as to whether the denture will be in harmony with the surrounding tissues and function properly in the mouth.

The upper residual ridge will become inwardly smaller according to the resorption of the alveolar bone. The clinician who thinks only about mechanical factors is afraid that the denture will be dislodged with a fulcrum on the ridge crest when the artificial teeth are placed buccally to it. This is the reason why the artificial teeth are arranged much more lingually to the position originally occupied by the natural teeth(Fig. 4). This leads to encroaching of the tongue space.

Incidentally, in patients who have been without dentures for a long time, regardless of missing teeth, or have been wearing small dentures, the tongue becomes enlarged due to muscular hypertrophy to take on or compensate for the reduced masticatory function[8]. It has also been reported that the muscle force of the tongue is stronger in the edentulous person than in the dentate person[26](Fig. 5).

As mentioned above, the tongue is larger and its muscle force is stronger in the edentulous person and thus the force of the tongue can not be neglected during teeth arrangement. In any situation, teeth should never be arranged lingually to the ridge. If the artificial teeth are arranged lingually, the pushing force of the tongue will be increased and the denture will be pushed outward. Even when the teeth are arranged with consideration of the leverage effect, contrary to expectations, the stability of the denture will be greatly diminished (Fig. 6). In addition, as tongue movement is inhibited, the functions of mastication and phonetics are impaired, with an increase in the feeling of having a foreign body in the mouth.

The alveolar crest, which is the basis of the interalveolar ridge line theory, can be easily located in

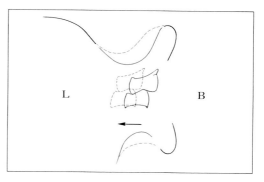

Fig. 4   The upper residual ridge becomes inwardly smaller as shown in Fig 3. If the artificial teeth are arranged on the ridge based on the mechanical theory, the artificial teeth will be placed inward more and more according to the resorption of the alveolar bone.

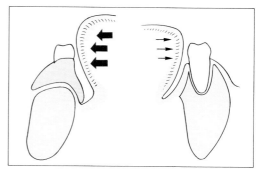

Fig. 5   The tongue is larger and its muscle force is stronger in the edentulous person than in the dentate person.

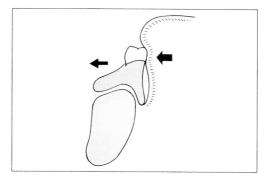

Fig. 6   If the teeth are arranged lingually, the increased force of the restricted tongue will push the denture out.

Problems of the interalveolar ridge line theory (3)

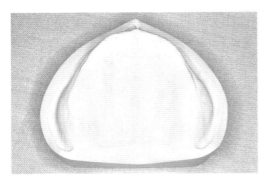

Fig. 7 The alveolar crest may vary a few millimeters depending on the clinician or it may have a wide range in the case of a favorable residual ridge.

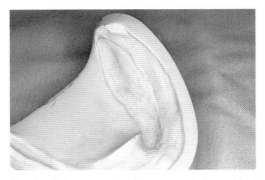

Fig. 8 If the resorption is severe and the residual ridge is flattened, the crest of the ridge can not even be guessed on the cast. Moreover, in the case of a concave ridge, no crest exists.

most cases with a favorable residual ridge. But sometimes even in the same case, it may vary a few millimeters depending on the clinician, or it may have a wide range(Fig. 7). On the other hand, when the resorption is severe and the residual ridge is flattened, the position of the ridge crest can not even be guessed on the cast. Moreover, in cases with a concave ridge, no crest exists(Fig. 8). In addition, the so-called alveolar crest on the cast and the crest of the alveolar bone or the mucosa with the lowest compressibility, thought to be the fulcrum of the lever system, do not always coincide[27](Fig. 9a, b). The interalveolar ridge line theory which is based on this vague reference may be questionable.

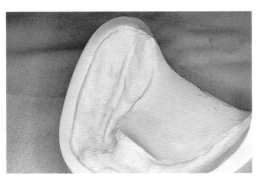

a

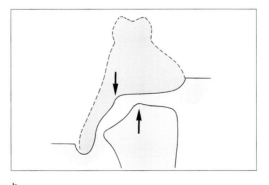

b

Fig. 9a, b   A cordlike elevation on the alveolar ridge may be thought to be the crest. The so-called alveolar crest on the cast and the crest of the alveolar bone which is thought to be the fulcrum of the lever system do not always coincide.

mony with the surrounding tissues.

The natural teeth are known to erupt in a place where the inward forces of the lips and cheeks are balanced by the outward forces exerted by the tongue(Fig. 4-2). Therefore, the movements of the surrounding tissues such as the cheeks and tongue, which greatly influence the position of the natural teeth, can not be ignored. After eruption, the natural teeth continue to be in harmony with the surrounding tissues in this position and also the cheeks and tongue continue to function properly. Therefore, if the artificial teeth occupy the same position as the natural teeth, the muscle balance between the buccal and lingual sides will be inherited and the dentures will be stable.

Similarly, the occlusal plane of the natural teeth is situated

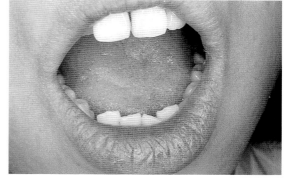

Fig. 4-2 The natural teeth erupt in a place where the muscle balance exists between the buccal and lingual sides.

The level of the occlusal plane (1)

As previously mentioned, if the occlusal plane is inclined toward the alveolar ridge, a shunting effect on the dentures will occur, causing a loss of denture stability(P. 51). The occlusal plane of the dentures shown in Fig.1, seems to be almost parallel with both the upper and lower alveolar ridges. However, it is obviously too low. Many dentures with such a low occlusal plane can be found.

Now, let us think why the occlusal plane has become so low in this case.

When determining the vertical level of the incisal edges of the anterior teeth using the occlusion rim, it is generally adjusted so that the upper anterior teeth are exposed about 1-2 mm below the border of the upper lip with the mouth slightly opened. Certainly, in this case, the central incisors are slightly visible and

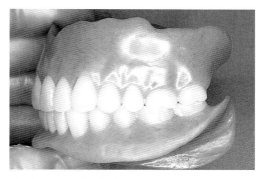

Fig. 1 The occlusal plane seems to be parallel with both the upper and lower alveolar ridges, however it is too low. When such dentures are seen, one should have the sense to think that"The upper denture is too large. It looks strange."

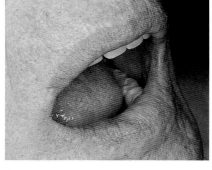 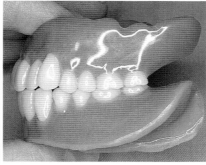 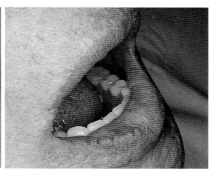

a   b   c

Fig. 2a～c When the dentures shown in Fig 1 are inserted, the central incisors are slightly visible and they look esthetically pleasing. However, the lower anterior teeth are covered by the lower lip and quite inferior to its border(a). The occlusal plane is raised up so that the incisal edges of the lower anterior teeth and the cusps of the lower first premolars are located at the level of the lower lip when the mouth is slightly opened. Thus the balance between the upper and lower denture is improved(b, c).

The level of the occlusal plane (2)

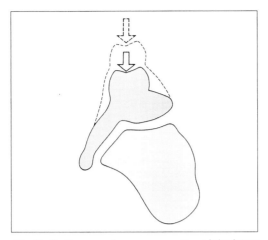

Fig. 3   In the case of severe resorption of the lower alveolar ridge, an attempt to improve the stability of the denture may be made by lowering the occlusal plane, that is, lowering the loading point of the occlusal force.

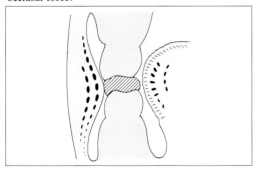

Fig. 4   The tongue brings the food onto the occlusal plane, then it holds the food between the upper and lower teeth by cooperating with the buccinator muscle so that the food can be easily crushed.

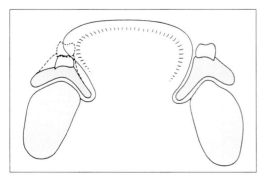

Fig. 5   When the artificial teeth are arranged too low, the tongue covers the low occlusal plane. Thus it can not bring food onto the occlusal plane, moreover it might be bitten during mastication.

thus appear to be esthetically pleasing(Fig. 2a ~ c). However, depending on the individual, the amount of upper tooth showing varies. Therefore if this level is adhered to, the entire occlusal plane will be affected, causing it to become either too high or too low. Turning our attention to the lower anterior region, the lower anterior teeth are covered by the lower lip and are quite inferior to its border. The incisal edges of the lower anterior teeth are located at the level of the lower lip when the mouth is slightly opened in most patients. Therefore there can be no doubt that the occlusal plane in this case is too low. The lower lip is said to be a better guide for the vertical orientation of the anterior teeth than the upper lip[9].

This may also result from an attempt to improve the lower denture's stability by lowering the occlusal plane, thus lowering the loading point of occlusal forces(Fig. 3). It sometimes happens as can be seen in a case with a unfavorable mandibular ridge such as this.

The function of the surrounding tissues, especially tongue function, during mastication in the dentate person, should be remembered. That is, the tongue brings the food onto the occlusal plane and then holds the food between the upper and lower teeth by cooperating with the buccinator muscle. The tongue presses the food outward and the buccinator presses it inward, so that the food does not escape and can then be easily crushed(Fig. 4). However, when the artificial teeth are arranged much lower than the occlusal plane of the natural teeth as in this case, even though the tongue tries to carry the food onto the occlusal plane, it can not perform this function because the tongue has already covered the low occlusal plane. Moreover, the tongue can not cooperate with the buccinator muscle in helping to crush the food, but will be bitten during mastication(Fig. 5). Therefore, the occlusal plane of the artificial teeth should be placed in the position where the occlusal plane of the natural teeth was situated, that is the functional level in which the cheek and tongue can cooperate to perform mastication smoothly.

harmoniously with the surrounding tissues for functional masticatory movements. Therefore the level of the occlusal plane of the artificial teeth should also be replaced similar to that of the dentate state. See "The level of the occlusal plane" for details.

If the artificial teeth are arranged in the position previously occupied by the natural teeth, the patient will become easily accustomed to this position because the tactile sensations from the tongue, cheeks and lips are not altered from that of the dentate state(Fig. 4-3). If the position differs too much from the previous position, the tactile sensation will be altered causing difficulty in speaking and eating. It does not need serious consideration, the lost teeth are simply replaced in their original position with artificial teeth.

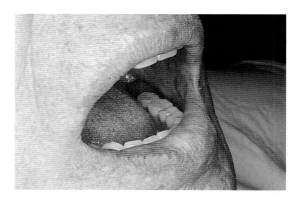

Fig. 4-3 If the artificial teeth are arranged as in Figure 4-2, the denture will be stable and also the patient will become quickly accustomed to the denture.

1. Selecting the anterior artificial teeth

The facial form of the patient should be classified into square, ovoid, or tapering. The form of the teeth should be in harmony with the form of the face; square teeth are used for those with a square face and so on. In addition, the patient's age, gender and personality should be taken into consideration when trying to improve the appearance. The color is also important; dark and opaque teeth should be selected for the elderly patient, light and translucent teeth for the young patient. The size of the teeth is selected by referring to the corner lines of the mouth recorded during jaw registration. Sometimes it may be necessary to modify the form and size of the artificial teeth. If the patient has existing dentures, the form, size, and color of the artificial teeth will be informative. In every case, the consent of the patient and any accompanying person must be obtained(Fig. 4-4).

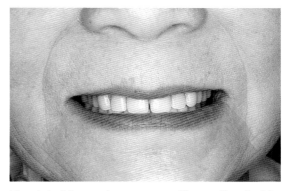

Fig. 4-4 Most patients seem to like small and white teeth. If these teeth are used, the appearance of the denture will be emphasized. Natural teeth are unexpectedly large and aged people have darker teeth.

2. Arranging the anterior teeth

1) The elderly appearance "caused by dentures"

As shown in Fig. 4-5, the prominence of the upper lip region is a characteristic feature of Japanese people. On the other hand, it is also characteristic that many patients wear dentures which make the upper lip region concave. If the upper lip is not adequately supported, the orbicularis oris muscle and its related muscles will not properly contract and thus the skin of the upper lip will lose its tension. Deep wrinkles and small vertical lines occurring on a skin which has already lost its elasticity emphasize the aging appearance. Moreover, the lips become thinner and the nasolabial fold changes direction to approach the corner of the mouth and the demarcation be-

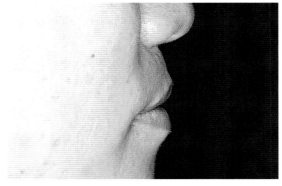

Fig. 4-5 The prominence of the upper lip region is a characteristic feature of Japanese people.

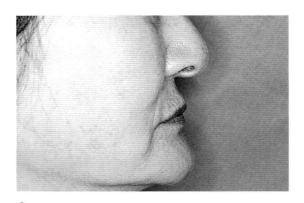 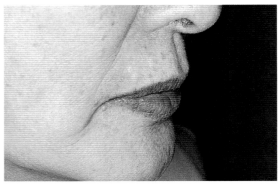

a   b

Fig. 4-6a   If the upper lip is not properly supported, its shape will be concave, thus the skin will lose its tension and wrinkles will occur, leading to the"denture-caused" elderly appearance. This is a characteristic feature of the denture wearing patient.

Fig. 4-6b   With a new denture having adequate upper lip support, the elderly appearance is no longer obvious.

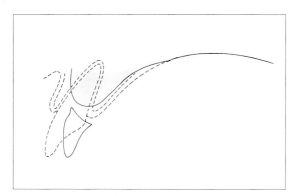

Fig. 4-7   The alveolar crest of the upper anterior region will move posteriorly according to the pattern of bone resorption. If this pattern is ignored and the artificial teeth are placed on the crest of ridge following the lever system theory, the lip support will be inadequate.

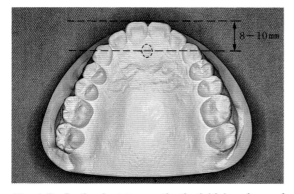

Fig. 4-8   In the dentate mouth, the labial surfaces of the upper central incisors are situated 8-10 mm in front of the middle of the incisive papilla. In addition, the incisive papilla lies on the line joining both canines.

tween the lips and cheeks becomes unclear. As a result, the patient has the so-called elderly appearance. As this is due to the denture, it should be called the elderly appearance "caused by the denture"(Fig. 4-6a, b).

In the upper anterior region, bone resorption following extraction will occur upward and inward because of the direction and inclination of the roots of the teeth and alveolar process. In addition, the buccal alveolar bone is thinner than that of the palatal side and thus bone resorption is faster and greater labially. Consequently, the alveolar crest will move posteriorly according to the resorption of the alveolar bone. Probably many clinicians ignore this bone resorption pattern and think that by placing the artificial teeth on the crest of the ridge, the lever system will be avoided, leading to stability of the denture. This is the reason why there are many dentures with inadequate lip support. However, this will not only make the esthetics worse but will also be the cause of poor denture retention and stability as mentioned later(Fig. 4-7).

For the provision of adequate and appropriate support of the lip, the artificial teeth must be placed in the positions occupied by the natural teeth.

2) Anatomical landmarks for the upper anterior teeth

The incisive papilla, which is almost stable in its position on the palate even after extraction, provides a good guide for seeking the horizontal position of the natural anterior teeth in the edentulous patient. As shown in Fig. 4-8, the labial surfaces of the natural upper central incisors are approximately 8-10 mm in front of the middle of the incisive papilla. In addition, the incisive papilla is also related to the canines and is situated on the line passing through the tips of the canines in

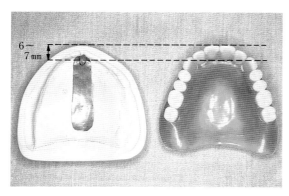

Fig. 4-9   As the incisive papilla moves forward and upward according to the resorption of alveolar bone, the labial surfaces of the upper central incisors should be placed 6-7 mm anterior to the middle of the incisive papilla.

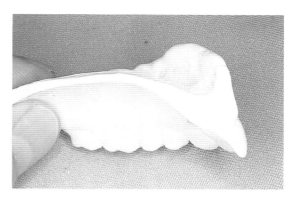

Fig. 4-10   In a case of severe alveolar bone resorption, if the anterior teeth are replaced in the natural tooth position, they might appear to stand a long way anterior to the ridge crest.

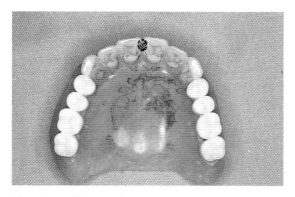

Fig. 4-11   The anterior teeth are arranged on the incisive papilla(shaded area). This pushes the molar teeth distally.

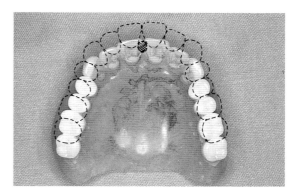

Fig. 4-12   If the artificial teeth are replaced in the natural tooth position by referring to the incisive papilla, the molar teeth will move forward and the tongue space will become wider.

the dentate person[28].

Therefore, the artificial anterior teeth can be placed to approach the natural tooth position by referring to the incisive papilla as a landmark. However, for clinicians who are not accustomed to this method, the artificial teeth may appear to stand a long way anterior to the residual ridge, especially in a case of severe resorption of the alveolar ridge(Fig. 4-9, 10). Also, clinicians who are afraid of leverage when the ridge acts as a fulcrum might be much more reluctant to follow this approach. However, it is just as important to set the anterior teeth in the natural tooth position and definitely will be the "key" for arranging all artificial teeth as well as restoring the esthetics. This will lead to a more successful complete denture.

As shown in Figure 4-11, sometimes a denture can be seen

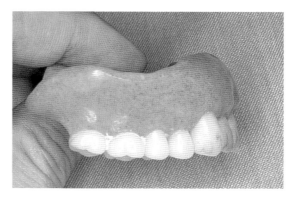

Fig. 4-13   This is a case in which the artificial teeth are arranged lingually. The polished surface of the labial flange seems to be protruded in order to remove the wrinkles of the upper lip, but this can not give proper and sufficient lip support.

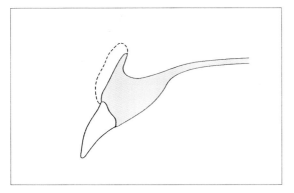

Fig. 4-14　If the impression of the width of the vestibule is not adequately recorded, proper contouring of the polished surface can not be created. Only the artificial teeth replaced in the natural tooth position seem to project forward.

with the anterior teeth arranged on the incisive papilla. In such a case, the lip can not be adequately supported and their position will also affect the arrangement of the molar teeth. The artificial teeth will be arranged altogether posteriorly and the tongue space will be greatly restricted. As shown in Figure 4-12, if the anterior teeth are placed in the position previously occupied by the natural teeth by referring to the incisive papilla as a landmark, the molar teeth will have an anterior shift accordingly and approach the position of the natural teeth. Thus the tongue space will become wider.

Among those cases in which the artificial teeth are arranged lingually to the natural tooth positions, the labial flanges of some dentures are thickened or protruded to provide tension to the skin of the upper lip, apparently trying to improve appearance(Fig. 4-13). However, if the artificial teeth still remain lingually, it will be difficult to restore the lip support and improve the appearance, even though the labial flange is thickened by waxing.

On the other hand, there are some cases in which the artificial teeth are almost arranged in the natural tooth position, but without an adequate impression of the labial vestibule, the proper contour of the labial polished surface can not be provided. Therefore only the artificial teeth seem to project forward(Fig. 4-14).

In the anterior region, as an extremely strong "facial seal" will be created by the lips and cheeks, even if the impression

Anterior teeth arrangement for more elderly patients

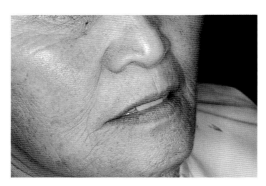

Fig. 1　For the more elderly patient, the anterior teeth should be arranged somewhat lingually being in harmony with the skin conditions of the other facial regions.

In the arrangement of the anterior teeth for more elderly patients, the amount of their protrusion should be considered. Nowadays, people live longer and even though they are called 'the elderly', they are still quite active. Therefore, it might be just enough to set the artificial teeth in the natural tooth position up to the age of seventy. However, almost all natural teeth are usually lost above the age of seventy. If the artificial teeth are arranged in their natural position to provide a natural appearance, only the skin surrounding the mouth will be tensed in the face. This will not be in harmony with the skin conditions of the other regions such as the wrinkles around the eyes. It looks somewhat unnatural, contrary to the objective of providing natural-looking dentures. In such cases, the teeth should be arranged somewhat lingually for producing an appearance such that others will get the impression like "Is it a denture? No, may be not...... Oh! it's a well made denture"(Fig. 1).

is inadequate and the flange is thin or short, the retention of the denture will still remain[7]. However, to join the denture border to the polished surface smoothly and provide a proper shape of the polished surface, a suitable impression of the width of the vestibule must be obtained.

3) Positioning the lower anterior teeth with respect to alveolar bone resorption

On a dentate lower cast(Fig. 4-15), it should be noted that the labial surfaces of the lower anterior teeth are situated anterior to the gingiva, alveolar mucosa and mucolabial reflection. Therefore in a lower denture, the labial surface of the anterior teeth must be situated anterior to the denture border located on the mucolabial reflection and also the shape of the labial polished surface must simulate that of the natural situation as much as possible(Fig. 4-16).

As most natural lower anterior teeth incline labially and the bone resorption after extraction occurs mostly on the labial side of the lower alveolar ridge as in the upper jaw, the crest of the residual ridge moves lingually following the resorption. Thus, in an edentulous case, the lower anterior teeth must be arranged labially to the so-called alveolar crest to replace the teeth in the natural tooth position. In a case with severe alveolar bone resorption, the teeth are arranged well above the labial sulcus which is far anterior to the crest of ridge(Fig. 4-17).

In some cases, as in Figure 4-18, the lower anterior teeth are arranged on, or even lingually to, the crest of the residual ridge regardless of the pattern of bone resorption. This might be the result of considering the leverage, but it will encroach

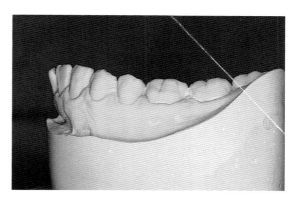

Fig. 4-15 In the natural dentition, the labial surfaces of the lower anterior teeth are situated anterior to the gingiva, alveolar mucosa and the mucolabial reflection.

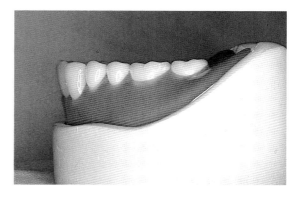

Fig. 4-16 Also in the lower denture, the labial surfaces of the anterior teeth should be situated anterior to the denture border and the shape of the labial polished surface must simulate that of the natural situation.

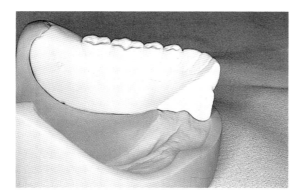

Fig. 4-17 In a case of severe alveolar bone resorption, the anterior teeth are arranged well above the labial sulcus which is far anterior to the ridge crest.

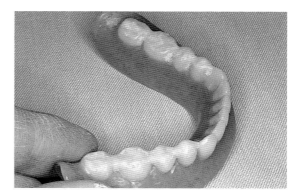

Fig. 4-18 If the lower anterior teeth are arranged on, or even lingually to, the ridge crest by considering the leverage, the tongue space will be encroached upon.

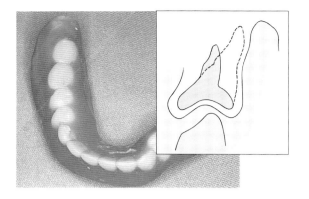

on the tongue space and the denture will be pushed out anteriorly by strong tongue forces which are increased by its compression. The shape of the labial polished surface will be completely different from that in the dentate state. It is shelf-like

Fig. 4-19 When the lower anterior teeth are arranged lingually, the shape of the labial polished surface becomes shelf-like causing disharmony with the movements of the lower lip.

Incision by the anterior teeth

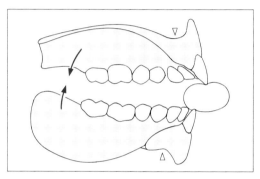

Fig. 1   When food is incised with the anterior teeth which have been arranged much more anterior to the alveolar crest, the posterior border of the denture is likely to drop easily due to the leverage with the fulcrum at the crest of the ridge. The antagonizing force is also small.

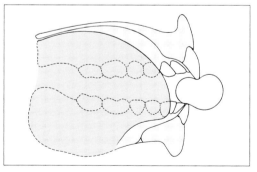

Fig. 2   While incising food with the anterior teeth, the upper denture is supported by the dorsum of the tongue and the lower denture is pressed downward by the tip and ventral surface of the tongue, leading to stability of the denture.

If the teeth are arranged by referring to the natural tooth position, the anterior teeth will be placed much more anterior to the alveolar crest. If food is bitten using these anterior teeth, the posterior border of the denture is likely to drop easily due to the leverage, with the fulcrum at the alveolar crest(Fig 1). The direction of the force applied when biting food with the anterior teeth is similar to that of removing the denture, so the antagonizing force is small. Thus, patients are instructed about the above mentioned mechanism and told not to bite with the anterior teeth.

However, patients do not seem to listen to things which may inconvenience them, and use the anterior teeth even though instructions to the contrary are given. It means that the dentures are being used without dropping unexpectedly.

Why does the denture not drop then? As incision is not performed like mastication and is carried out consciously, the patient can control the magnitude and direction of the force during biting, and thus they are somewhat able to resist the dislodging force of the denture[9]. In addition, as shown in Figure 2, when denture wearers become accustomed to dentures, during biting, they seem to support the upper denture by the dorsum of the tongue and press the lower denture downward using the tip and ventral surface of the tongue. This will enhance the stability of the dentures. However, the anterior alveolar ridge, which can not tolerate excessive force, shows increased bone resorption when pressure is applied, thus it is better not to use the anterior teeth for incising.

and is not in harmony with the movement of the lower lip-(Fig. 4-19). The shelf-like flange may be caused by arranging the upper anterior teeth too far lingually. Therefore, it can be solved by checking again the arrangement of the upper anterior teeth and rearranging them in the natural tooth position as mentioned previously.

3. Overlap of the anterior teeth

The anteroposterior relationship of the upper and lower anterior teeth, that is the horizontal overlap, is automatically decided by the relation between the upper and lower residual ridges as described previously. But generally, it seems that no attention is paid to this because there are many dentures which have the upper and lower anterior teeth arranged in contact. Also, a certain overlap is given to some dentures by only considering the occlusal balance regardless of the relation between the upper and lower residual ridges.

The upper and lower anterior teeth should not be in contact in the centric occlusal position in any case(Fig. 4-20a, b). Settling of complete dentures occurs 1-2 weeks after insertion, mainly due to the compression of the mucosa under the denture base. So, if the anterior teeth are arranged in contact, following the settling of the dentures, an impact between the opposing anterior teeth and an upward thrust of the anterior region will occur during occlusion, leading to an earlier loss of denture retention(Fig. 4-21a~d). Even in a case where the amount of the denture settling is small in the early stages, when the alveolar ridges resorb later and the occlusal vertical dimension is decreased, an impact and upward thrust will also occur in the anterior region causing the loss of denture retention. In addition, due to the excess pressure exerted, resorption of the alveolar ridge in the anterior region will be increased and soft tissue hyperplasia, that is so-called flabby gums, will occur in this region.

In the case where the natural upper and lower anterior teeth were not in contact in the centric occlusal position, the artificial teeth need not, and must never be in contact on the dentures. Even if they were in contact in the natural dentition, they should be arranged so as not to be in contact for the above mentioned reasons. In such cases, the author tries to avoid any contact of the opposing anterior teeth by arranging the lower anterior teeth somewhat lingually. If this is done, the position of the lower artificial teeth will be a little different from that of the natural teeth and thus the esthetic appearance will be occasionally somewhat sacrificed. However, the teeth should be arranged out of contact just enough to

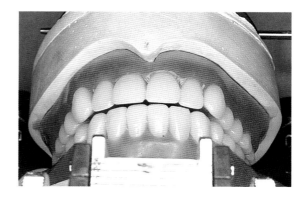

a

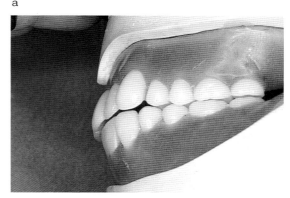

b

Fig. 4-20a, b The upper and lower anterior teeth should not be in contact in the centric occlusal position. Even though the teeth were in contact in the natural dentition, they should be arranged out of contact at least just enough to compensate for the amount of settling after insertion.

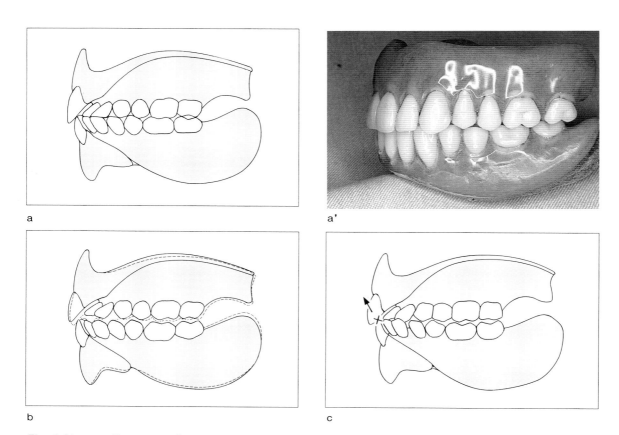

a

a'

b

c

Fig. 4-21a~c Denture settling occurs 1-2 weeks after insertion mainly due to the compression of the mucosa under the denture base(b). If the anterior teeth are arranged in contact(a, a'), following settling of the denture, an impact and upward thrust will occur in the anterior region during occlusion(c), and denture retention will be lost.

compensate for the amount of settling which occurs soon after insertion. By providing such a horizontal overlap, the incisal guide inclination is reduced and then there will also be an improvement in the stability of the complete denture.

As mentioned above, it is important to arrange the anterior teeth in a position as close as possible to that of the natural teeth, for both esthetics and function. But in the case of maxillary or mandibular protrusion, special consideration is required (See "Tooth overlap in patients with maxillary or mandibular protrusion").

As many edentulous patients have a small sagittal condylar guide inclination, the vertical overlap should not be deepened as in the natural state, to achieve denture stability. In other words, an overlap should be provided, in which impact between the anterior teeth can be avoided. If impact occurs, denture retention and stability will be compromised. It is thought that protrusive balance is not so important during mastication, as this is performed mainly by lateral movements.

Tooth overlap of patients with maxillary protrusion (1)

In patients who had an Angle's Class II, division 1 malocclusion in their natural dentition, in order to provide a good appearance, it is not uncommon for the upper anterior teeth to be arranged more lingually than their normal position and sometimes even some of the alveolar process is removed to arrange the teeth further back. In this way, the prominent appearance is removed and the appearance of the patient is apparently improved. However, if one sticks to arranging the teeth posteriorly, the tension of the upper lip will be lost and a youthful appearance may disappear. Also, a deep vertical overlap of the anterior teeth and a marked forward translation of the mandible during function are characteristic of these cases(Fig. 1a, b). If this is neglected and the anterior teeth are arranged posteriorly, the horizontal overlap will reduce and the large mandibular movement during function will be hindered. The dentures may be displaced by the anterior teeth impacting during function(Fig. 2a, b).

Therefore, in order to improve the appearance of those patients with maxillary protrusion without loss of denture retention, a method is used in which the upper anterior teeth are arranged at a higher level than the natural teeth without altering their anteroposterior position. Thus, the deep vertical overlap is reduced, leading to improvement in the facial appearance and a smoothing of the mandibular movements. In some cases,in addition to lifting the teeth, the teeth have to be arranged a little more posteriorly for the improvement of the appearance. In such cases, the upper and lower anterior teeth should be adjusted to greatly reduce the vertical overlap. It is important to give a shallow incisal guide inclination for good denture stability(Fig. 3a~g).

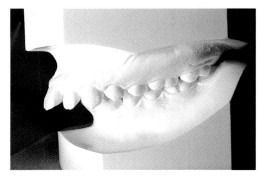

a

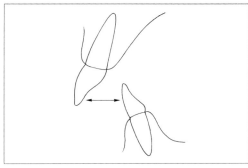

b

Fig. 1a, b Patients having maxillary protrusion are characterized by a deep vertical overlap of the anterior teeth and a marked forward movement of the mandible.

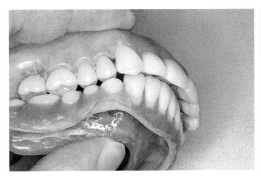

a

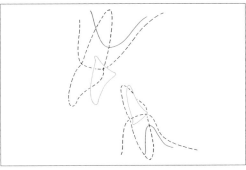

b

Fig. 2a, b If the anterior teeth are arranged posteriorly just to improve the appearance, the horizontal overlap will become small, and large mandibular movements will be hampered. Thus the dentures will be displaced by anterior tooth contact during function.

Tooth overlap of patients with maxillary protrusion (2)

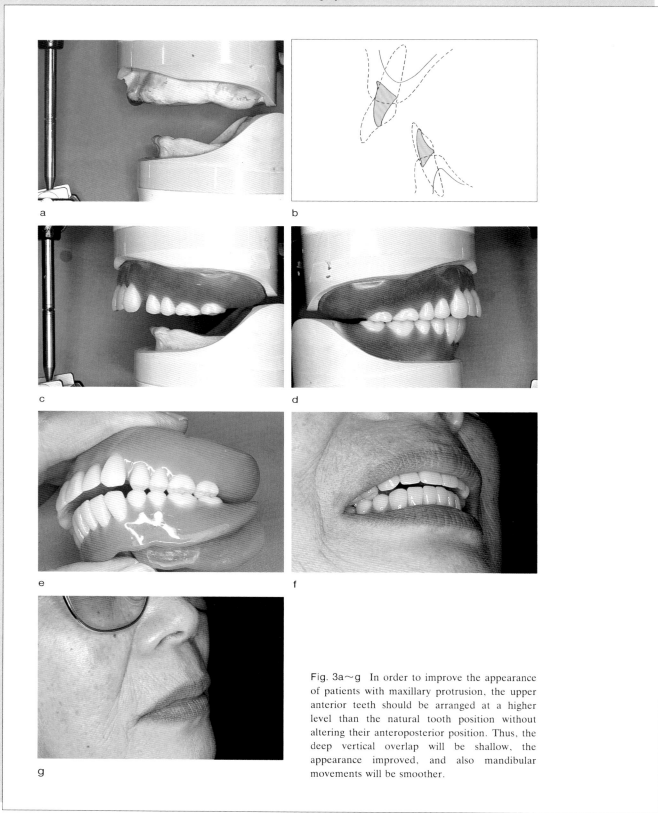

Fig. 3a~g In order to improve the appearance of patients with maxillary protrusion, the upper anterior teeth should be arranged at a higher level than the natural tooth position without altering their anteroposterior position. Thus, the deep vertical overlap will be shallow, the appearance improved, and also mandibular movements will be smoother.

Many patients with mandibular protrusion have a marked translation of the mandible during function, similar to those patients with maxillary protrusion. Therefore, even though the appearance of the patient can be improved as much as they expect, the upper anterior teeth should not be arranged to cover the lower anterior teeth regardless of a marked mandibular movement and the relationship of the upper and lower residual ridges(Fig. 1a, b). In patients with mandibular protrusion, arranging the teeth in an edge-to-edge-like incisal relationship(the upper and lower anterior teeth are not in contact) is the limit. However, if only the upper anterior teeth are proclined to produce an edge-to-edge relationship, the inclination will become steep and consequently the prominence of the chin will be undesirably exaggerated. Thus, when the anterior teeth are placed in an edge-to-edge relationship, if possible, the upper anterior teeth should be arranged more labially than their natural position(Fig. 2a, b). However, for this purpose, it is essential that the impression of the labial vestibule is made as wide as possible and then the border of the labial flange is thickened adequately. As a patient with mandibular protrusion has a marked sunken upper lip and poor tension in this region, it is effective to adequately support the upper lip in this way. As a result, the maxillary deficiency in the dentate state will be considerably improved. However, in those patients with a very large discrepancy between the upper and lower jaws, it is considered that the appearance may not sufficiently be improved by dentures.

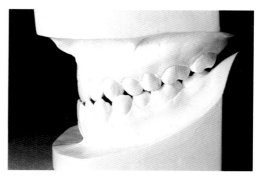

a

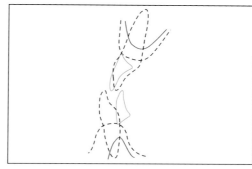

b

Fig. 1a, b In the case of mandibular protrusion, the lower anterior teeth are frequently arranged further lingually to produce a "normal" relationship, but the impact of the opposing anterior teeth will easily occur due to the marked translation of mandible during function.

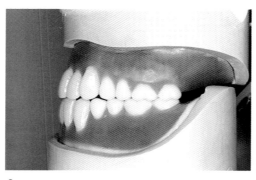

a

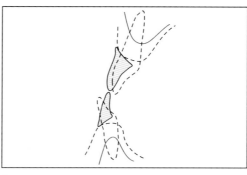

b

Fig. 2a, b In the case of mandibular protrusion, the anterior teeth should be arranged in an edge-to-edge-like relationship. If possible, the upper anterior teeth should be arranged more labially than their natural position.

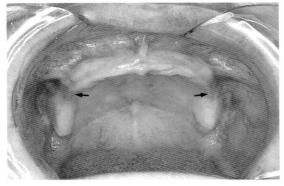

a

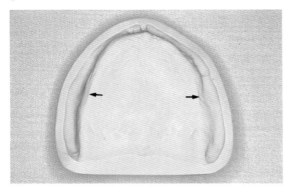

b

Fig. 4-22a, b   The remnants of the lingual gingival margins of the natural teeth are seen as a cordlike elevation of mucosa near the crest of the residual ridge. The positions of the natural teeth can be guessed by this location.

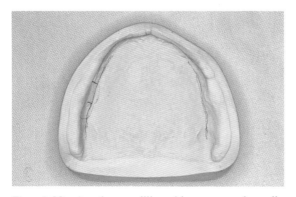

Fig. 4-23   As the cordlike ridge moves buccally according to the alveolar bone resorption, it is necessary to arrange the posterior teeth so as to sit partly on this elevation in order to bring the artificial teeth close to the position of the natural teeth.

4. Arranging the posterior teeth

1) Anatomical landmarks for the upper posterior teeth

When imagining the position occupied by the natural upper posterior teeth in the edentulous situation, the remnants of the lingual gingival margins are recommended as a good landmark, buccolingually. Watt found that a cordlike elevation of mucosa situated near the crest of the residual ridge is the remnant of the lingual gingival margin of the natural teeth by placing tattoo spots on the mucosa before extraction (Fig. 4-22a, b). He suggested that the position occupied by the natural teeth can be guessed by using this location as a guide[8].

However, this remnant of the lingual gingival margin moves 2-4 mm outward according to the resorption of the residual ridge, thus by reducing this amount, the position occupied by the natural teeth must be guessed. In other words, in order to bring the artificial teeth close to the natural tooth position, the posterior teeth have to be arranged so as to sit partly on this cordlike ridge. To what extent the artificial teeth sit on the remnants of the lingual gingival margin is decided by considering the amount of alveolar bone resorption.

2) The pushing effect of the cheeks

When the artificial posterior teeth are placed in the position occupied by the natural teeth, they would be arranged much more buccally to the so-called alveolar crest, especially in a case of severe bone resorption (Fig. 4-24a, b). Those who believe that the alveolar crest is the fulcrum of leverage will be concerned that this arrangement may cause denture dislodgment or even denture fracture.

Now, we should pay attention to the cooperative effects of the tissues surrounding the denture during masticatory movements, especially the role of the cheeks and tongue.

Regarding the inward pressure of the cheek, if the artificial teeth are arranged lingually to the natural tooth position by considering the alveolar crest, the buccinator muscle which can not act cleverly like the tongue will not be able to approach the artificial teeth, leading to a lack of inward pressure of the cheek. As a result, the outward pressure of the tongue will not be balanced by the inward pressure of the cheek. The reduction of inward pressure will lead to a loss of the peripheral seal and thus denture retention will be reduced and also food will easily enter into the vestibule. To improve the retention and stability of the denture by appropriately utilizing the inward pressure of the cheeks, the artificial teeth should be arranged where the natural teeth were situated (Fig. 4-25).

be arranged where the natural teeth were situated(Fig. 4-25). If they are arranged in the natural tooth position, even if the food is held on one side, the peripheral seal will be maintained because the buccinator muscle will effectively exert pressure against the resulting polished surface on the opposite side. Thus the dislodgment of the denture caused by the leverage at the fulcrum on the residual ridge will be inhibited on the balancing side. This phenomenon acts as a retainer for the denture. On the working side, while the strong center fibers of the buccinator muscle are holding the food in cooperation with the tongue, the muscle can simultaneously exert a strong upward and inward force against the denture. This inward pressure will inhibit the denture tilting caused by the leverage at a fulcrum on the alveolar crest(cheek's pushing effect) and thus dislodgment and fracture of the denture will never occur (Fig. 4-26).

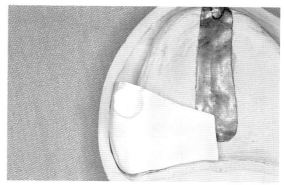

a

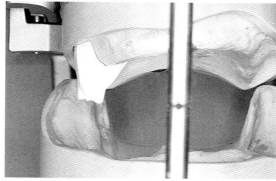

b

Fig. 4-24a, b When the artificial teeth are placed where the natural teeth were, they will be arranged much more buccally to the alveolar crest, especially in the case of severe bone resorption.

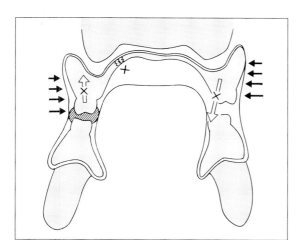

Fig. 4-26 When the artificial teeth are arranged in the natural tooth position, even if food is held on one side, the peripheral seal will be maintained by the effective inward pressure of the cheek on the opposite side, thus dislodgment of the denture will be inhibited. On the working side, the buccinator muscle holds food and simultaneously exerts a strong force against the denture which will inhibit the denture tilting caused by any leverage(cheek's pushing effect).

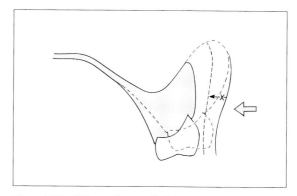

Fig. 4-25 When the artificial teeth are arranged lingually, the buccinator can not approach the artificial teeth, leading to a lack of inward pressure of the cheek. As a result, the peripheral seal will be lost and thus the retention will decrease(solid line). To appropriately utilize the cheek's inward pressure, the artificial teeth should be arranged in the position of the natural teeth(dotted line).

The importance of the impression of the buccal space

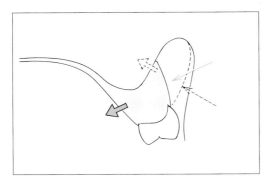

Fig. 1   If the artificial teeth are arranged in the position of the natural teeth on a cast in which the buccal sulcus was recorded narrower than its actual width, the buccal polished surface will face upward and outward. Thus, the inward pressure of the buccinator muscle would act to displace the denture(solid line). If the width is appropriately recorded, the polished surface will face downward and outward, thus the pressure of the buccinator muscle will improve the retention of the denture(dotted line).

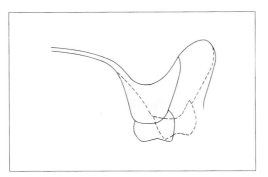

Fig. 2   When a narrow impression is recorded and another more appropriate impression is not prepared, the only place where the artificial teeth can be placed is on the residual ridge.

When the artificial teeth are arranged in the position of the natural teeth, it is important to make an appropriate impression of the vestibule with the aim of restoring the missing tissues to the pre-extraction situation. Among them, the impression of the upper buccal vestibule is the most critical. When the buccal space is broad, such a broad impression must be made and then the flange of the denture should be also thickened.

Even if the artificial teeth are arranged in the position of the natural teeth, if the impression of the buccal sulcus was recorded narrower than its actual width, the buccal polished surface of the resulting denture will not be appropriate as shown in Fig. 1 and the denture will be easily displaced. In addition, as the artificial teeth are located outside the denture flange, cheek biting will easily occur. Thus, when a cast made from such a narrow impression is prepared, clinicians would think that arranging the artificial teeth in the position of the natural teeth is a terrible mistake. They just rely on the residual ridge as something to refer to and would probably arrange the artificial teeth on the residual ridge following the interalveolar ridge line theory etc.(Fig. 2). Firstly, it is important to make an appropriate impression because only then can we replace the artificial teeth in the position of the natural teeth. As mentioned before, if one has knowledge of the anatomy and physiology regarding the tissues surrounding the denture, using appropriate impression materials, it may be possible to make an excellent impression. Thereafter, the movement of the muscles can be captured as a friend, not an enemy.

3) Anatomical landmarks for the lower posterior teeth

Regarding the anatomic landmarks used for locating the positions of the lower molar teeth, Pound reported that the lingual surfaces of the lower molars are situated between two lines projected from the buccal and lingual aspects of the retromolar pad to the mesial aspect of the cuspid[29](Fig. 4-27). Also, as stated by Ortman, the lingual cusps of the natural molars are approximately in vertical alignment with the mylohyoid ridge and thus the mylohyoid ridge is a reliable guide for determining the lingual limit of the artificial lower posterior teeth. The lower posterior teeth must never be arranged lingually to this ridge[30](Fig. 4-28). Both are generally used as guides to guess the position occupied by the natural teeth. However, in the former case, the standard lines will be changed according to the position of the canine which has been arranged previously. For example, if the lower anterior teeth are arranged on or lingually instead of labially to the alveolar ridge, the Pound line will also be placed more lingually to that of the natural dentition. Also in the latter case, it may be difficult to identify the position of the mylohyoid ridge on a cast. So, attention must be paid to the application of these guides.

The author arranges the posterior teeth almost in the center of the posterior denture-bearing area, buccolingually(Fig. 4-29). However, for this purpose, the external oblique ridge and mylohyoid ridge must have been recorded in the impression as the buccal and lingual landmarks respectively, as mentioned before. When this position is verified using guides such as the Pound line and mylohyoid ridge, it is found to be almost the same as that of the natural molar teeth.

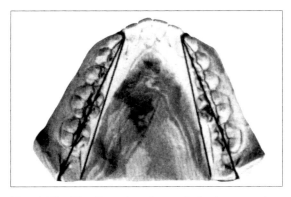

Fig. 4-27 The lingual surfaces of the lower molars are situated between two lines projected from the buccal and lingual aspects of the retromolar pad to the mesial aspect of the cuspid(Pound, E).

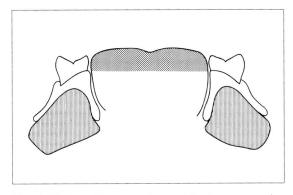

Fig. 4-28 The lingual surfaces of the lower posterior teeth are never lingual to a vertical line extending from the mylohyoid ridge(Ortman, H.R.).

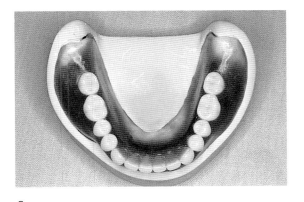 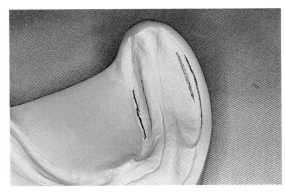

a   b

Fig. 4-29a, b The posterior teeth are arranged almost in the center of the posterior denture-bearing area buccolingually on the cast containing both the buccal and lingual landmarks, the external oblique ridge and mylohyoid ridge. The position of the artificial teeth may seem to be rather buccal.

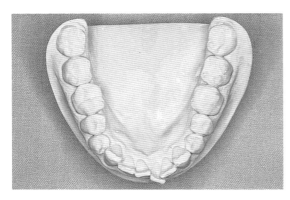

Fig. 4-30　In the molar region of the lower natural dental arch an undercut tends to occur lingually and its degree increases as the dental arch is followed posteriorly.

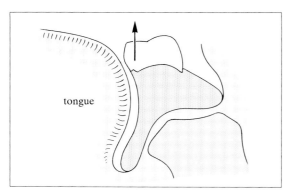

Fig. 4-31　If the posterior teeth are arranged in the position where the natural teeth were, the undercut will also occur on the lingual polished surface under the teeth. The tongue will bulge into the undercut and raise the denture.

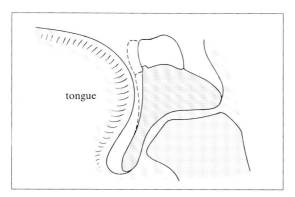

Fig. 4-32　If posterior teeth which are narrow buccolingually are used, no undercut will occur lingually under the teeth.

In addition, when the lower posterior teeth are placed where the natural teeth were situated, one has to also consider the size of the artificial teeth. An undercut tends to occur increasingly under the lower molars of the natural dental arch as it is followed posteriorly(Fig. 4-30). So, also in the denture, if the artificial teeth are arranged in the position occupied by the natural teeth, an undercut will be produced on the lingual polished surface under the posterior teeth. Thus, the tongue will bulge into the undercut and raise the denture, causing it to be dislodged(Fig. 4-31). However, as is generally known, the occlusal surface area of the artificial posterior teeth is smaller than that of the natural teeth in order to reduce the load on the supporting tissues during mastication. This will also work effectively in this situation. The use of posterior teeth which are narrow buccolingually will produce no undercut under the teeth as shown in Fig. 4-32. More favorably, these teeth are also smaller mesiodistally, so that the position of the posterior teeth shifts mesially where there is less undercut in the natural dentition(Fig. 4-33). By using artificial teeth which are much smaller than the natural teeth, a large tongue space can be obtained. In addition, the forces from the cheeks and tongue will be balanced. So, this situation can resolve problems arising in edentulous patients, who typically have a large, strong tongue.

Sometimes patients complain "The denture is too big." The reason is not that the denture itself is big, but more commonly, the artificial teeth are arranged lingually so the tongue space is restricted. Therefore, in the case of such a complaint, the denture should be checked by referring to the above mentioned guides(Fig. 4-34a, b).

Practically, the upper and lower artificial teeth should be

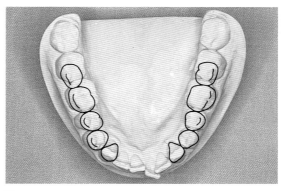

Fig. 4-33　As the artificial posterior teeth are smaller mesiodistally, the position of the posterior teeth shifts mesially where there is less undercut in the natural dentition.

placed firstly following the guides mentioned above, then the teeth adjusted a little, so that harmony can be achieved between the upper and lower teeth.

It should be noted that the premolars, as with the anterior teeth, are arranged buccally to the alveolar crest(Fig. 4-35).

4) Arranging the premolars and the modiolus

At the corner of the mouth situated almost in the position of the lower first premolar, many muscle fibers of the muscles of mastication and expression such as the buccinator and orbicularis oris converge to form a muscle knot called the modiolus. When the buccinator, the orbicularis oris, etc. contract during functional movements such as mastication or speech, the modiolus strongly pushes the buccal side of the premolar region. Some consider that this muscle pressure serves as the retention force for the upper complete denture by holding up the buccal cusps of the premolars, but for the lower denture, if the buccal side of the premolar region is widened as in the molar region, the tension of the modiolus will push out and dislodge it. Fish[31] suggested to narrow the lower denture in the premolar region to prevent a collision with the modiolus. This means arranging the artificial teeth more lingually to that position previously occupied by the natural teeth and trimming the border of the buccal flange(Fig. 4-36). But this suggestion is a somewhat questionable.

The buccinator, which contracts during mastication, can produce an effective muscle contraction only if its anterior and posterior ends are fixed. Its anterior end is at the modiolus which is supported by the first premolar. Therefore, if the first premolar is placed more lingually to the position of the natural teeth, the buccinator will lose its support during function and can not function effectively during mastication as in the dentate state. The buccinator holds food between the molar teeth with the cooperation of the tongue, prevents its escape from the corner of the mouth when it slides forward along the inclined occlusal plane, and returns it to the occlusal surface of the molar region by peristaltic movements[5]. To perform these functions smoothly, the first premolar should be arranged in the position of the natural teeth, namely buccally to the alveolar crest. So as to withstand the strong inward muscle pressure against the denture, a concave shelf should be provided properly on the lingual polished surface as will be mentioned later. By providing this shelf, the denture resistance will be enhanced and denture retention will not be diminished(refer to P. 103).

In addition, if the support from the artificial teeth is inadequate in the region of the corner of the mouth, not only

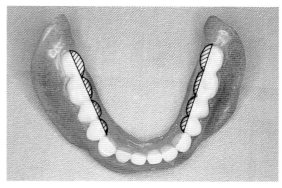

a

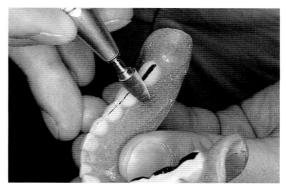

b

Fig. 4-34a, b a: A denture with the complaint, "The denture is big and my mouth is filled with the denture." b: As the tongue space was restricted, the lingual cusps of the artificial teeth were trimmed and the tongue space was widened. This procedure made the denture feel less bulky and more stable.

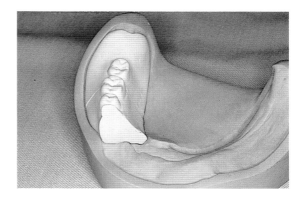

Fig. 4-35 The premolars are arranged buccally to the alveolar crest like the anterior teeth.

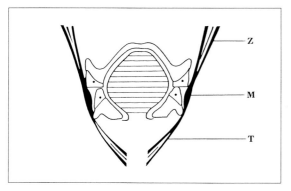

Fig. 4-36   The narrow arch of the lower denture in the first premolar region keeps it clear of the modiolus(M)(Fish, E.W.).

the functions of the lips and cheeks but also those of the muscles of expression will be disturbed and facial expressions can not then be properly performed. Also considering this factor, adequate tension should be provided in the region of the corner of the mouth as in the dentate situation.

The resorption of the alveolar ridge and the denture contour (1)

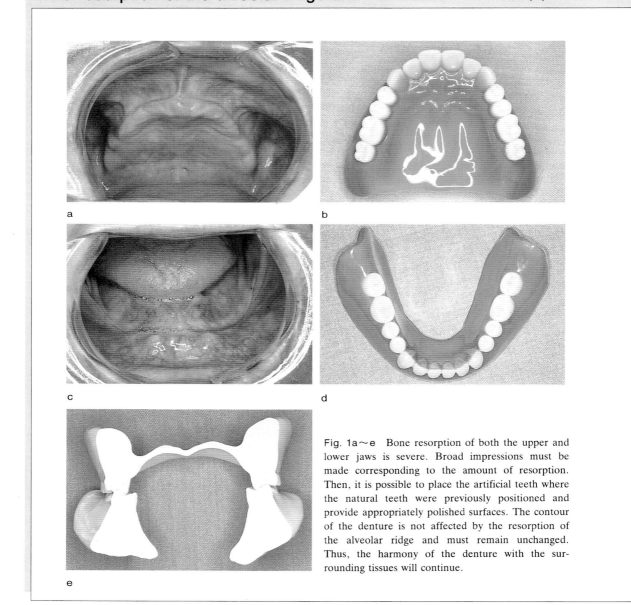

Fig. 1a~e   Bone resorption of both the upper and lower jaws is severe. Broad impressions must be made corresponding to the amount of resorption. Then, it is possible to place the artificial teeth where the natural teeth were previously positioned and provide appropriately polished surfaces. The contour of the denture is not affected by the resorption of the alveolar ridge and must remain unchanged. Thus, the harmony of the denture with the surrounding tissues will continue.

In order that the denture may be harmonious with the surrounding tissues and function by appropriately harnessing muscle movements, not only the position of the artificial teeth but also the contour of the denture should not be changed regardless of the progress of alveolar bone resorption(Fig. 1a~e). In other words, the resorbed alveolar ridge should be compensated for by the denture base during denture fabrication. Figure 2 shows a cross section of the alveolar ridge with a denture in place. The denture contour is not affected by the resorption of the alveolar ridge. It must remain unchanged and only the same amount of denture base resin as that of bone resorption will be added on the impression surface.

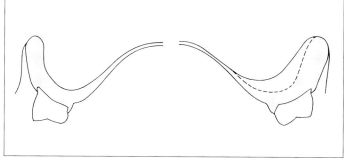

Fig. 2 Even if alveolar bone resorption progresses, only resin of the denture base will be added on the impression surface corresponding to the amount of resorption. The position of the artificial teeth and the contour of the denture must not be changed.

Which is the better material for artificial posterior teeth, resin or porcelain?

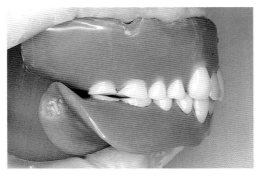

a

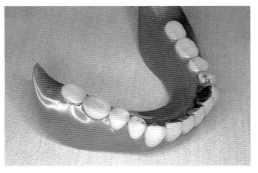

b

Fig. 1   As the resin teeth wear away rapidly, the occlusal vertical dimension will decrease in a short time, leading to collision of the anterior teeth and occlusal disharmony. It is necessary to check the occlusion regularly.

It is difficult to cut our fingers with a plastic sheet, but easy with a piece of glass, even with little effort. Without giving this example, it is well known that porcelain teeth are superior to resin teeth in their ability to cut, crush and grind as well as being abrasion resistant. It has been reported that masticatory efficiency is greatly decreased when porcelain teeth were replaced with resin teeth in the case of complete dentures[32]. However, porcelain teeth are rarely used in general practice. This is because patients prefer resin teeth, and dentists like using it.

If a significant error is found in the occlusion, when resin teeth are used, the occlusion can be corrected easily and rapidly by grinding the teeth. Even when the error is so great that it can not be corrected by grinding, the occlusal surface of the resin teeth can be built up with self-curing acrylic resin, and the centric occlusal position can then be correctly obtained using the patient's jaw as an articulator(p. 117).

However, as resin teeth tend to wear away rapidly with food, in the most severe case of rapid wear, the occlusal vertical dimension will decrease in six months to one year after insertion of new dentures. To make matters worse, together with the resorption of the alveolar ridge, collision of the opposing anterior teeth and an occlusal disharmony will occur, leading to ill-fitting dentures.

In cases where the centric occlusal position can not be easily obtained or the dentures are easily moved due to unfavorable ridges, it is obligatory to use resin teeth because the occlusion can be easily corrected. But even in such cases, porcelain teeth are still recommended for use on either of the jaws. Just as with a chopping board and a kitchen knife, when using something for cutting on one side, one can expect to improve the masticatory efficiency. If possible, the occlusal surfaces of the resin teeth should be replaced with metal after occlusal correction.

Section 5

Try-in of the dentures

Try-in of the dentures

The artificial teeth have been arranged according to the outlined principles on the occlusion rims contoured at the jaw registration appointment. These wax trial dentures are then inserted into the mouth and checked for esthetics and function. Some modifications are carried out so that they fit the patient more accurately.

Generally, the try-in procedure for checking the arrangement of the artificial teeth is divided into two steps, one for the anterior teeth and another for the posterior teeth. If these two steps are performed simultaneously, time and labor will be wasted. When the position of the anterior teeth has to be greatly altered, the posterior teeth will also have to be rearranged in relation to the shift of the anterior teeth. At the try-in for the anterior teeth, the appearance can be improved by making the trial denture suit the personality of the patient and also by modifying it according to the patient's wishes. For the posterior teeth, only the occlusion can be checked roughly, but the occlusal contacts, phonetics, etc. can hardly be checked because the wax dentures move easily. Tests for denture retention and stability are out of the question. After the try-in procedure for the anterior teeth, the author performs the arrangement of the posterior teeth and then carries out a rough waxing procedure. During the try-in procedure for the posterior teeth, the outline of the denture base and the form of the polished surface are merely checked. If there is enough time, final checking of the position of the gingival margins of the anterior teeth and the interdental papillae is done for esthetic purposes.

Try-in for the anterior teeth arrangement

The average life span has become longer and it seems that the requirements of elderly patients for esthetics nowadays are much stronger as they might be thinking "Life is short, so let's live everyday to its fullest". If dentures which make the patient look young are inserted, the patient will have a more positive attitude when acclimatizing to the new dentures, even if a little pain is experienced. In the case of a new denture, if the patient just keeps it in his/her mouth for a reasonable period of time(until the next appointment), it is likely to be successful. The area where a sore-spot is situated can be clearly recognized. Therefore providing a pleasing appearance may be a shortcut to success.

However, as mentioned previously, the anterior teeth are generally arranged a long way posterior to the position occu-

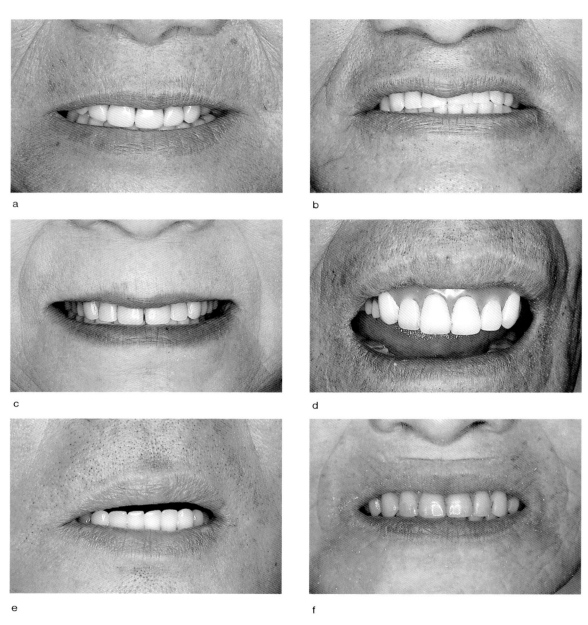

a

b

c

d

e

f

Fig. 5-1a∼f   Common errors in anterior teeth arrangement. a: The center line is off to one side. b: Edges of the anterior teeth are in line and the occlusal plane is inclined. This gives an artificial appearance. c: The artificial teeth are too small and white. d: The upper anterior teeth are arranged too low and a large amount of the gingiva(denture base) is exposed during smiling. e: The lower anterior teeth are too visible when slightly opening the mouth. The occlusal plane is too high. f: The support for the upper lip is inadequate producing the elderly appearance.

pied by the natural teeth and this is a ringleader causing an elderly appearance in many dentures. Therefore, if the artificial teeth are positioned where the natural teeth were previously situated, the patient will think that (s)he looks younger. There is no need to consider any difficult procedure, only if the artificial teeth are arranged in the same position as that of the natural teeth, will patients be satisfied with the appearance(Fig. 5-1a~f).

The positions of the individual teeth are also affected by the preference of the clinician. However, when the anterior teeth are set in an irregular fashion, care must be taken not to arrange them too irregularly. For example, such irregularities might mean the imaginary roots of the artificial teeth would interfere with each other and should be avoided because this never appears in nature(Fig. 5-2). If the patient has a photograph taken when (s)he had her/his own natural teeth, it will be helpful at the try-in. Although the teeth can not be seen on the photograph, the appearance and contours of the lips and the lower part of the face can be grasped.

On the other hand, in order to construct a denture that contains the patient's heart and desires, approval by the patient should be obtained at the try-in appointment for the anterior teeth. However, it is a tough job. Even though approval was obtained during the try-in, if the patient goes home with new dentures and a comment is made by a fussy daughter such as "Oh mother, you look older", the denture will be quickly put into a pocket and all effort will have been in vain. During the try-in, the patient is given the opportunity to observe the arrangement of the anterior teeth using a mirror, but in this way, it is difficult to grasp the three-dimensional image. If the patient looks at her/himself in two mirrors held against each other, this may be a little more effective.

Anyway, it seems very difficult for patients to evaluate the appearance of the denture by themselves. It may be an idea to observe the appearance together with another family member at the try-in appointment because the main people who complain about the appearance of the denture are not the patients themselves.

In a successful case with a comment like "Oh mother, you look younger", the author is astonished at the changes in patient's clothes, make-up and even behavior at the next visit. To receive this type of pleasure, the author makes an effort to provide a good appearance for his patients.

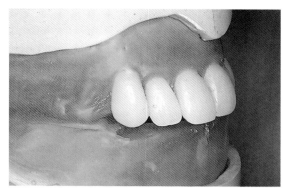

Fig. 5-2 The imaginary roots of the artificial teeth (lateral incisor and canine) would interfere with each other. These irregularities never appear in nature and should be avoided.

Section 6

Designing the polished surface

Designing the polished surface

The polished surface of a denture consists of the labial, buccal, lingual, and palatal parts of the denture base and the outer surfaces of the artificial teeth except the occlusal surfaces. But this surface is not so popular as the other two surfaces of the denture, namely the impression surface and the occlusal surface and its significance has not been widely recognized. However, the retention of the denture is greatly affected by the quality of the shape of the polished surface. Wilfred Fish who termed it the polished surface emphasized that if the polished surface is appropriately contoured and in harmony with the movement of the surrounding tissues such as the cheeks, lips and tongue, the movements of these muscles can be utilized for the retention of the denture, and not cause its dislodgment[31](Fig. 6-1). Brill et al. proved that the activity of the surrounding muscles appreciably improves the retention of the denture. In addition, he suggested that in cases with an unfavorable residual ridge, this muscle activity which presses the denture in place is much more important than the other denture retention factors[33].

Since this polished surface adjoins the occlusal surface of the artificial teeth and the impression surface of the denture base, it can, of course, be greatly affected by the positions of the artificial teeth and the denture border, that is, the impression of the denture-bearing area determining the border. The polished surface is molded during waxing. Therefore, if the previous steps such as artificial teeth arrangement and/or impression making have not been suitably performed, the polished surface can not be properly molded due to the limitation of these steps, in spite of the utmost effort during waxing.

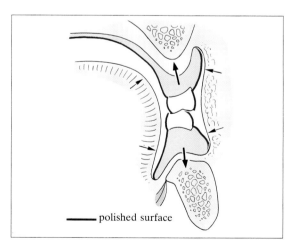

——— polished surface

Fig. 6-1 The polished surface of a denture consists of the labial, buccal, lingual, and palatal parts of the denture base and the outer surfaces of the artificial teeth except the occlusal surfaces. Whether the movements of the surrounding muscles can be applied for denture retention depends upon the quality of the polished surface.

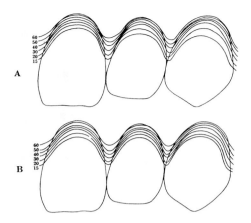

Fig. 6-2   Clinical crown forms at different ages. A: male, B: female (Matsumoto, N.).

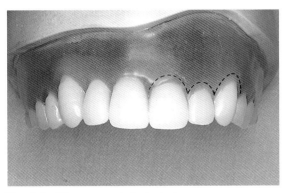

Fig. 6-3   The unreceded gingival margins like those of young people should be contoured properly (dotted line).

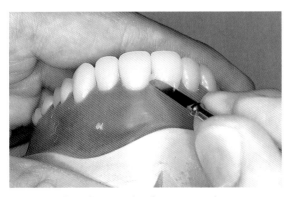

Fig. 6-4   Prominences in the root regions are not necessary. The appearance of the neck regions which are visible during smiling is important.

1. Waxing in the anterior region

Waxing of the anterior region is considered essential for good denture esthetics, but the author thinks that it is adequate when the height of the gingival margins is correct. In the dentate person, the gingival margin recedes with aging[34](Fig. 6-2). Nevertheless, many dentures are commonly seen, having similar gingival margins to those seen in young people, in other words, showing little recession (Fig. 6-3). Especially when the interdental papilla of a denture is high and sharp, it looks unnatural and thus it is easy for others to notice that dentures are being worn. Of course, the height of the gingival margin depends on age, but it should be formed so that at least the finish lines on the necks of the artificial teeth can be seen.

Generally, on the labial polished surface, providing prominences by adding wax on the area corresponding to the imaginary roots of the artificial teeth is considered necessary to improve the esthetics. Sometimes, the prominences and depressions on the polished surface are shaped more markedly than those in the dentate state. This unevenness is not necessary for esthetic improvement, and will only lead to the accumulation of food. If the teeth are arranged so that a large area of the contoured gingiva is exposed, one should not be too proud of the esthetics. This appearance is unnatural because the gingivae do not appear so large in the dentition.

Moreover, to further improve the appearance, some clinicians perform stippling on the gingiva or embed vessel-like fibers in the gingiva. However, as only small parts of gingiva are visible, even when smiling, waxing in this region is time-consuming and is not overly effective. The only real value of this artistic waxing is to make the patient feel satisfied with the appearance of the denture when it is outside the mouth.

Creating a root prominence for each individual tooth is not necessary. However, a slight eminence should be formed all over the flange, starting from the necks and eventually blending into the denture border. Above the canine tooth, a large eminence is shaped for lip support by referring to the appearance. The author always takes great care concerning the appearance of the neck region which is visible when smiling (Fig. 6-4). Needless to say, any unevenness is not necessary and the interdental papilla should be carved high and sharply in the posterior region, since this is not an area of great esthetic concern.

The polished surface and the flange technique (1)

The flange technique is a well-known method to functionally determine the arch form of the artificial teeth and the contours of the polished surfaces so that they will be in harmony with the movements of the surrounding tissues. In this technique, the neutral-zone, that is, an area where the inward pushing forces of the lips and cheeks are neutralized by the outward forces of the tongue, is located using the functional movements of the lips, cheeks and tongue situated in contact with the dentures. The polished surface is molded, and the artificial teeth are arranged in this zone[35-37].

However, even this method is not perfect. The neutral zone will vary greatly according to the patient's ability to follow the instructions of the functional movements, a difference in the functional movements instructed by different operators or further errors in softening the wax(Fig. 1a ~ c). Therefore, it is also necessary to have a mental image of the appropriate polished surface in order to decide the quality of the polished surface molded by this method. In actual fact, while performing the flange technique, the operator usually compares the formed polished surface with its mental image and repeats functional modification of the parts that are different from the image to gradually bring the form closer to the proper polished surface(Fig. 2).

Now, if all the procedures of the flange technique are properly performed and the polished surface is functionally formed, whether it can be used just "as it is" should be considered.

In other words, we have to consider whether or not the polished surface functionally formed to adapt to the existing muscle movements is the most appropriate for the new denture. The muscle pressure is not appropriate in many patients because the tissues surrounding the dentures may not function properly. Enlargement of the tongue and inward bulging of the buccal mucosa can be frequently seen, which seems to have occurred due to not wearing dentures for a long time or wearing small dentures. Therefore, just the form molded by muscle pressure can represent an individual difference of the present oral situation, but it can never indicate what form it should essentially possess.

The molded polished surface must be modified so that the surrounding tissues will recover their original form and pressure, and the retention and stability of

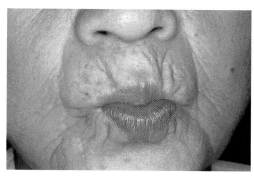

a

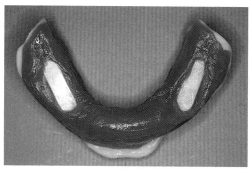

b

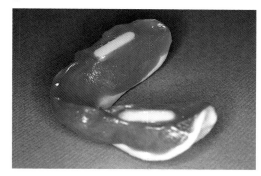

c

Fig. 1a ~ c The neutral zone is located with soft wax by the patient's functional movements. However, the neutral zone is varies greatly according to the patient's ability to perform the functional movements, a difference in the movements instructed by different operators, or errors in softening the wax.

The polished surface and the flange technique (2)

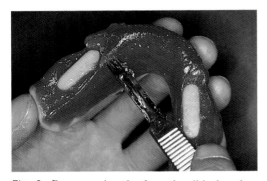

Fig. 2   By comparing the formed polished surface with its mental image, the parts that are different from the image are functionally modified step by step to bring them closer to the appropriate form. For this procedure, one must have the mental image of an appropriate polished surface.

the denture will then improve.

On the other hand, "prosthetics" literally means to supply artificial substitutes for missing tissues and to restore the former condition, including the functions of the surrounding tissues. However, in clinical practice, it is important to decide to what extent one has to restore the original situation. With aging, patients lose their teeth and also control of their temporomandibular joints and muscles. Thus, the masticatory system is deprived of mutual cooperation. Therefore, by considering these factors, artificial teeth arrangement and the form of the polished surface should be modified so that they are in harmony with each condition and enhance the activity of the surrounding tissues.

In any case, it is important to firstly completely comprehend "What was the original situation." On this basis, by considering "it is a denture", it is essential to construct a prosthesis possessing a form adaptable to the present situation.

2. The buccal polished surface of the maxillary denture.

Refer to "The importance of the impression of the buccal space"(P. 84).

3. The lingual polished surface of the mandibular denture

If the impression of the lingual border is extended adequately and additionally, the occlusal vertical dimension, the level of the occlusal plane, and the size and positions of the artificial teeth are correct, a concave form(concave shelf) can be made on the lingual polished surface as shown in Figure 6-5a, b. Regarding the impression, if it is not adequately extended beyond the mylohyoid ridge, the large polished surface necessary to place the concave shelf will not be obtained, and even with improvisations in the laboratory, the proper shape cannot be produced. When an appropriate concavity is provided on the lingual polished surface during waxing, two fingers can be placed on the shelves of the completed denture as shown in Figure 6-6. Even if one attempts to push the denture upward by the other hand, the denture can still be held by the fingers placed on the shelves. In the mouth, as the tongue will ride on the shelves instead of the fingers, the denture can be securely seated in position because of the outward and downward pressures of the tongue actively pressing the shelves towards the alveolar ridge(Fig. 6-7).

When inserting the new dentures, dentists seem to frequently use the words "You will soon get used to the dentures". It is appropriate to use these words when a device such as the concave shelf is prepared and in fact the words mean "You will soon become accustomed to handling the device". However, it is irresponsible to say "You will soon get used to the dentures" with the thought of imploring the patient to get used to them without making the device on the denture. If a concave shelf is provided and its role is explained to the patient using the fingers as shown in Figure 6-6, they will quickly become used to handling the denture. If only the tongue is placed on the shelves, the denture will not be dislodged, even though the mouth is opened wide. When the patient can prevent the denture from being dislodged using the tongue, the patient will be confident in wearing the denture and make a serious effort to master its handling.

By the way, if the concave shelf is just provided blindly when the artificial teeth are arranged lingually or large artificial teeth are used, an undercut will occur under the lingual surfaces of the teeth. The tongue will slip into this undercut

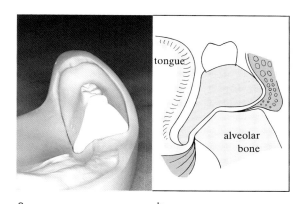

a b

Fig. 6-5a, b If the impression of the lingual border is adequately extended and the occlusal vertical dimension, the level of occlusal plane, and the size and positions of the artificial teeth are all appropriate, it is possible to make a concave shelf on the lingual polished surface.

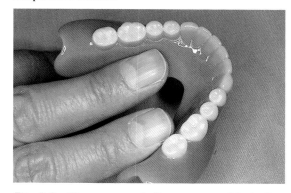

Fig. 6-6 The concave shelf serves as a "device" to stabilize the denture. Even if one tries to push the denture upward by the other hand, the denture can still be held by the fingers placed on the shelves. In the mouth, the tongue will ride on the shelves instead of the fingers.

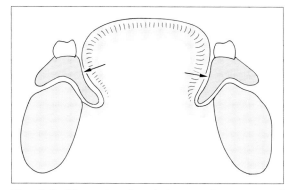

Fig. 6-7 The outward and downward pressures of the tongue press the shelves actively towards the alveolar ridge, thus the denture can be firmly seated in position.

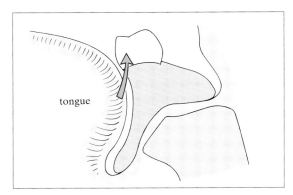

Fig. 6-8   If the concave shelf is provided when the artificial teeth are arranged lingually, an undercut will occur under the lingual surfaces of the artificial teeth. The tongue will slip into this undercut and push the denture upwards.

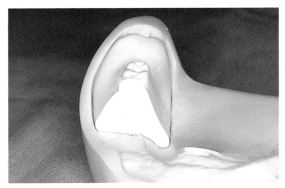

Fig. 6-9   The buccal polished surface of the mandibular denture should be contoured so it is slightly convex or straight.

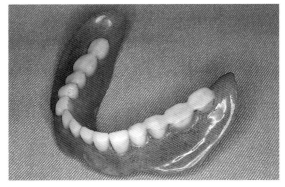

Fig. 6-10   The buccal polished surface of the mandibular denture is generally made concave.

and push the teeth upwards, thus the application of the concave shelves to this situation will worsen the stability of the denture(Fig. 6-8). When an undercut occurs under the lingual surfaces of the teeth, it is a signal to rearrange the artificial teeth more buccally or to switch to smaller ones. If the concave shelf is properly formed, this means that impression making, jaw registration, and selection and arrangement of the artificial teeth have been correctly performed. Therefore the quality of the form of the concave shelf is a good indicator for judgement of the quality of the previous procedures.

4. The buccal polished surface of the mandibular denture

Contrary to the lingual polished surface of the mandibular denture, the buccal polished surface is contoured slightly convex or straight(Fig. 6-9).

Generally, it is thought that the buccal polished surface must be made concave in this region so as to direct the muscle forces exerted on the polished surface towards the alveolar ridge and then use them for denture retention, by referring to the direction of the buccinator and the shape of the muscle bundles. This is widely carried out in clinics (Fig. 6-10). However, the middle and lower fibers of the buccinator differ in the degree and direction of contraction during function. Therefore, if the form of the polished surface is molded without considering the degree of contraction during function, the resultant form can not conform to the shape of the tissues in action.

If the buccal polished surface of the mandibular denture is made concave as shown in Figure 6-10, when the patient eats sticky food such as biscuits, the biscuits will collect and adhere to the concave part because the buccinator can not press firmly against this concavity(Fig. 6-11a). The food not only adheres to the denture but also accumulates in the buccal sulcus and further wedges under the denture base, causing pain during mastication or dislodgment of the denture. In fact, the form of the adhered biscuits indicates the proper contours of the polished surface. Therefore a convex form is essential to avoid this condition(Fig. 6-11b). A convex form in this region bulges somewhat more than that in the dentate state. Regarding its anatomical background, the explanation of the buccal pouch by Fish[31] is easy to understand. The author would like to explain it by quoting some of Fish's explanation.

As shown in Figure 6-12, during mastication in the dentate person, the food is held in place by the buccinator pressing it inwards and the tongue pressing it outwards so that it can be easily crushed between the teeth. After the food is crushed, half of it falls into the cheek and the remainder comes onto the tongue. The bolus of food on the tongue is pushed back between the teeth by the tongue and crushed again. This process will be repeated without interfering with the action of the buccinator in the presence of the food in the buccal sulcus. As the lower fibers of the buccinator are weak and flaccid, these form a space like a pouch(pocket) which can be filled with food. So, the strong middle fibers of the buccinator can still hold food without any interference, despite the presence of food in the sulcus and continuing mastication. This pouch can be also seen in the monkey. When the monkey is given a large amount of food all at once, its cheeks will immediately bulge to temporarily store the food in the cheek pouches(Fig. 6-13). Therefore, the buccal polished surface should be molded in a convex shape to fit into this pouch. So, the action

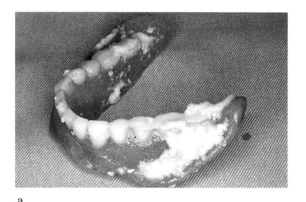 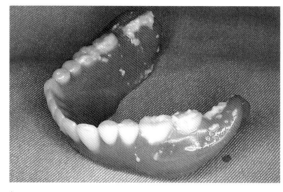

a   b

Fig. 6-11a, b   a: If the buccal polished surface is molded into a concave shape, food will collect and adhere to the concave part because the buccinator can not press firmly against this concavity. b: In a new denture with a convex form, no food adheres to the surface.

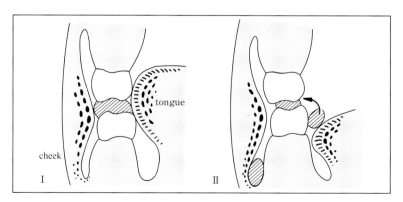

Fig. 6-12   I; The food is held between the buccinator(its middle fibers) and the tongue, and crushed. II; The bolus of food falls buccally and lingually. The bolus of food which comes onto the tongue is pushed back between the teeth and crushed again. This process is repeated in the presence of the food in the buccal sulcus.

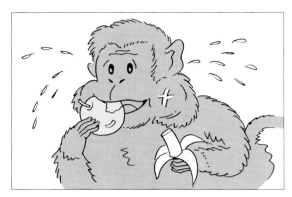

Fig. 6-13　When a monkey is given a large amount of food at one time, it will temporarily store the food in the cheek pouches and continue to eat with bulging cheeks.

of the buccinator during mastication will not be interfered with and furthermore, the muscle can press firmly against the denture in this weak muscle fiber region because of its convex form, leading to an improved peripheral seal and a reduction in food accumulation.

At first some patients may feel a little uncomfortable with this convex form which protrudes a little more than that in the dentate state. In such a case, as mentioned by Fish, if the necessity of the form for denture retention and stability is explained and then the convex part is thinned down a little one week later, the discomfort will be reduced. At this time, it is important to make as much noise as possible during grinding of the convex area, so only a small amount of grinding will be neccessary.

Incidentally, if the impression making of this region has not been performed adequately by referring to the external oblique ridge, molding the convex polished surface in the buccal pouch will be difficult(Refer to P. 23, Fig. 2-7).

Section 7

Correcting the occlusion

Correcting the occlusion

After processing, according to the index grooves made in the base of the cast, the casts with dentures are remounted on the articulator in the same position as before curing(Refer to "Split-cast method", P. 61). The correction of the occlusion is then performed on the articulator. The occlusal errors due to changes that may occur during processing are corrected and furthermore the occlusal surfaces are ground so that they are in harmony with the mandibular movements.

The retention of a complete denture prosthesis can not be expected to be so great, since it just rides on the mucosa. Therefore, to maintain the stability of the dentures, a bilaterally balanced occlusion is generally applied so that the upper and lower teeth can be in balancing contact wherever they occlude(Fig. 7-1). However, once a bolus of food is held between the upper and lower teeth on one side, the teeth on the opposite side will be separated(Fig. 7-2). Therefore, in this occlusal scheme, it may be said that the upper and lower teeth can obtain a balanced occlusion and the denture can be stabilized only when no food is in the mouth. The dentures can not be balanced during the movements of mastication which are, of course, the most important. However, if a balanced occlusion is provided, the dislodgment of the denture can certainly be prevented during nonfunctional movements such as bruxing and clenching or when food is finely ground during mastication. So, we can not say that this occlusal scheme is valueless. However, as the upper and lower teeth are separated during most of the masticatory process, it can not be the most important factor for ensuring recovery of masticatory function.

In any case, a lot of time is needed to establish a bilaterally balanced occlusion on the articulator and moreover occlusal adjustment in the mouth is extremely difficult as the compressibility of the mucosa differs from region to region. Generally, occlusal correction may not be adequately understood. There are many dentures in existence, whose occlusion

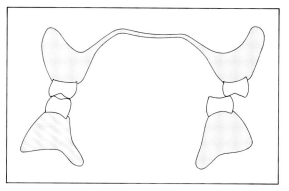

Fig. 7-1　In a complete denture for which very good retention can not be expected, a bilaterally balanced occlusion is generally applied to maintain denture stability.

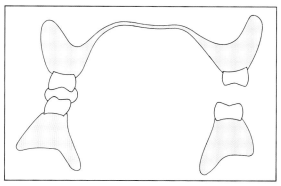

Fig. 7-2　Even if a bilaterally balanced occlusion is provided, once a bolus of food is held between the upper and lower teeth, the teeth on the opposite side will separate. The dentures can not be balanced during mastication.

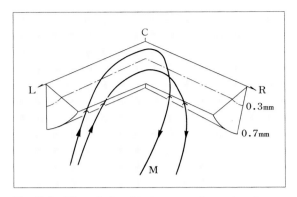

Fig. 7-3   The relationship between the paths of masticatory movement and lateral movement(Ai, M.). At the terminal stage of mastication its path is close to that of the lateral sliding movement(within 0.7 mm) and the length is about 2 mm in the molar region(C: centric occlusal position, CL,CR: lateral movement path, M: masticatory movement path).

is hardly adjusted or the cusps are markedly reduced by grinding.

Ai precisely examined the sliding movements during mastication and reported that the path of sliding movements seen at the terminal stage of mastication almost coincided with that of the lateral sliding movements with no food in the mouth and its length was about 2 mm in the molar region. He mentioned that the masticatory movements were influenced by cuspal inclination and directed into the centric occlusal position[23,38] (Fig. 7-3). The important point in occlusal correction lies in this zone.

Section 8

Denture insertion and subsequent oral examinations

Denture insertion and subsequent oral examinations

Although the behavior of the tissues around or under the denture vary in a complicated fashion during function, the impression is only a record of one static condition. The denture, which is constructed on the basis of such a record, can not be compatible with the surrounding tissues that change infinitely during function. Of course, the denture is designed and adjusted by considering these dynamic factors, but there is a limit. Moreover, when the dimensional changes of the denture base resin during polymerization are also taken into consideration, the situation becomes more complicated. Therefore, during insertion, adjustment of the borders and the impression or fitting surface of the denture is required so that these will fit the movements of the tissues during function. Particularly, when the impression is made by a nonpressure impression technique, it is necessary to examine the contact between the mucosa of the denture-bearing area and impression surface under load and relieve pressure spots that may be caused by occlusal forces. Similarly, it is essential to examine the occlusion in the mouth at the insertion appointment and then eliminate any premature contacts and cuspal interferences or any other problems so that the dentures can adapt well to the mouth.

Since the denture settles a little after insertion due to occlusal pressure, the fit of the denture and the occlusion will change. Therefore, it is necessary to perform fine adjustments in response to these changes until the denture is perfectly seated. Serious problems may not occur after insertion if the design of the denture and all procedures are performed correctly. However, should there be some trouble, to prevent this from becoming serious, it is essential to examine the fit of the denture the next day after its insertion.

On the other hand, patients tend to think that they can eat anything with their new dentures just after insertion. Instructions should be given not to eat hard foods at first and to gradually learn how to chew by beginning with soft foods.

Fabrication of dentures with passing grades(1)

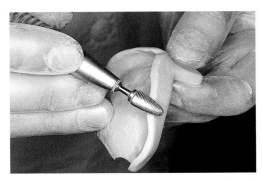

Fig. 1 Check the individual tray in the mouth and reduce all peripheries to be about 3 mm short of the tissue reflection.

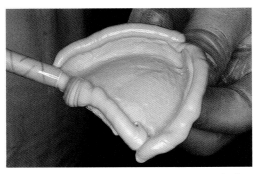

Fig. 2 Place heavy bodied type elastomeric impression material along the periphery of the tray. A silicone impression material(Hydroflex heavy body, GC) is used in this case.

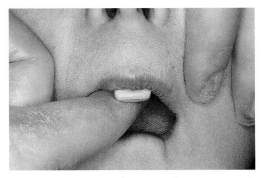

Fig. 3 Instruct the patient to perform movements such as sucking a finger or pursing the lips. Simultaneously, the dentist assists border molding by massaging the lips and cheeks gently with his/her hand.

In the fabrication of a complete denture, many steps such as impression making, jaw registration, artificial teeth arrangement, molding the polished surfaces and occlusal corrections are continuous with no interval, and make those clinicians who are not confident in denture construction want to avoid these steps if possible. To construct a functional denture which will work well in the mouth, it is best if every step is followed perfectly. However, since this is not easy, it may be better to make an effort to improve one step in the procedure, and by doing so, improving the overall quality of the denture. In the case of denture fabrication, even if the overall quality of work at every step is very high, if one step is a failure, the denture will not be functional. On the other hand, even though the quality of the work done in all the steps is barely adequate, if no step in the procedure was a failure, it could become a "usable denture".

Here the author would like to mention several methods of impression making and jaw registration which are more user friendly than the usual methods and can make one obtain at least a pass mark in denture fabrication.

1) A simple method of impression making to obtain a pass mark

A common procedure for impression making of an edentulous jaw is to first make an individual tray on the study cast obtained from the preliminary impression. The borders are then molded with modeling compound sticks and finally an impression is completed with an impression material that flows easily.

In actual fact, one can obtain a precise impression by these consecutive steps, but this is a very difficult technique for beginners. Moreover, as it takes a lot of chairtime, complete denture patients, who are mostly elderly, will become physically fatigued. In order to reduce the fatigue, it may be thought to construct a denture using a simple impression such as an alginate impression made with a stock tray. However, if such a simple technique is used, the completed denture, in many cases, will not be adequate during function, since border molding which records the mobilities of the muscles in function can not be performed. Anyway, an essential step during impression making is molding the borders with an individual tray.

However, regarding border molding, as mentioned by Levin[7], many dental students only remember that

Fabrication of dentures with passing grades (2)

they have spent too much time doing incomprehensible work with modeling compound sticks during clinical training. Most of them seem to be firmly determined not to touch modeling compound any more after graduation. Furthermore, older dentists may encourage them with kind suggestions that this procedure is not necessary.

A convenient method is to use a heavy bodied type of elastomeric impression material for border molding[39,40] (Fig. 1 ~ 6). In this method, the border extensions are determined by the mucosa, not by the clinician. However, the procedure can be done with relative ease and it is also possible to obtain a reasonable impression. There is no doubt that one can get a pass mark in impression making by this method, so it is hoped that the dentist grasps a mental image of the outline of the denture base by repeating this method and then proceeds to an advanced level, that is, "making the impression based on the mental image".

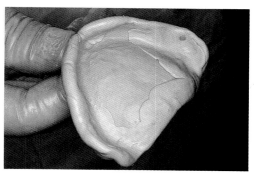

Fig. 4   The completed maxillary border molding. The elastomeric impression material which flowed into the inside of the tray is removed.

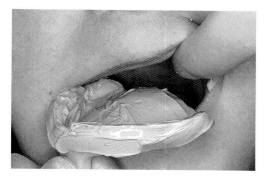

Fig. 5   The final impression is completed with light bodied type elastomeric impression material. A new silicone material developed by the author's research group is used in this case.

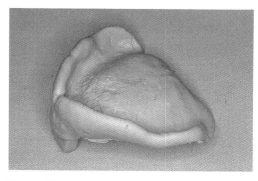

Fig. 6   The final maxillary impression completed with an elastomeric impression material.

Fabrication of dentures with passing grades (3)

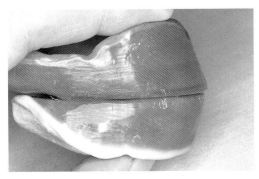

Fig. 7   Determine the occlusal vertical dimension by the method shown on p. 52.

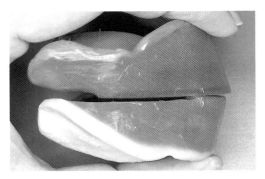

Fig. 8   Remove 2 mm of the upper part of the lower occlusion rim distally to the canine area.

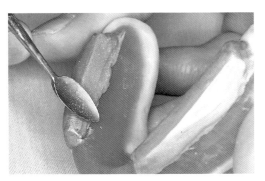

Fig. 9   Add Aluwax on the cut out part.

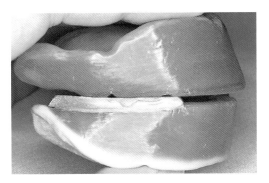

Fig. 10   Add Aluwax to a height of 3 mm above the occlusal plane.

2) Jaw registration to obtain a pass mark

For those who never want to use a gothic arch tracer, the following method is recommended to obtain a pass mark in jaw registration.

(1) By replacing the upper part of the lower wax rim with Aluwax(Aluwax Dental Products Co. Michigan), it becomes possible to soften the wax evenly, thus the displacement of the wax rims during recording will be minimal[39](Fig. 7～14). The use of a water bath is essential for this method.

(2) There is also one method where the denture is firstly completed using resin teeth, and when it is inserted, if there is a large error in occlusion, the occlusal surface is built up with self-curing resin to correct the occlusion(Fig. 15, 16). In this way, a denture that properly fits the mucosa is used for recording and the occlusion can therefore be easily corrected. However, the self-curing resin will wear rapidly, so it would be better to replace the occlusal surfaces with metal after occlusal adjustment.

Fabrication of dentures with passing grades (4)

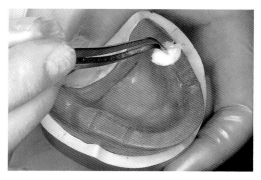

Fig. 11   Cut two V-shaped notches in the posterior region of the upper occlusion rim and coat them with vaseline.

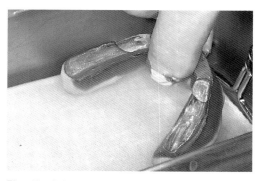

Fig. 12   Soften the Aluwax in a 125°F(51°C) water bath to obtain the best working consistency.

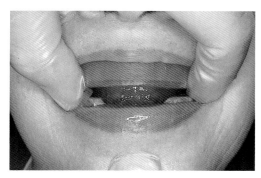

Fig. 13   Record the centric occlusal position. The unremoved part of the wax rims in the anterior region serves as a good guide to determine the occlusal vertical dimension

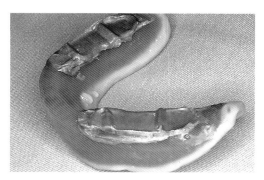

Fig. 14   Chill the wax record under cold running water.

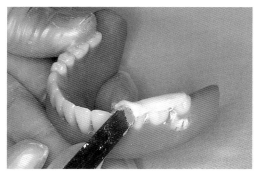

Fig. 15   Add tooth-colored self-curing resin on the posterior occlusal surfaces of the mandibular denture.

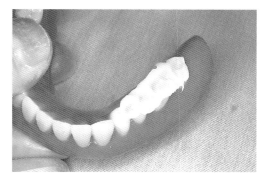

Fig. 16   When the patient closes the mouth with the mandible guided to the centric occlusal position, the occlusal surfaces of maxillary posterior teeth are recorded in the resin. Trim the resin to reestablish the contours of the teeth.

Section 9

Clinical procedure

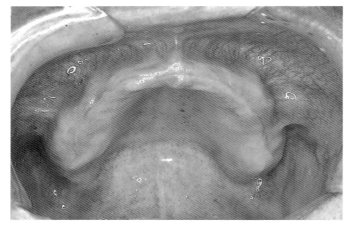

Fig. 9-1　A mental image of the outline of the denture base should be created by referring to the anatomical landmarks. An intraoral examination should be completed not only by glancing at, but also by closely observing and palpating the alveolar ridge.

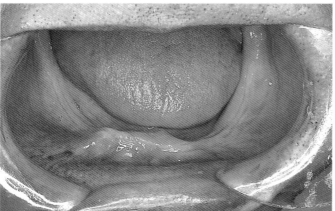

Fig. 9-2　When searching for the locations of the external oblique ridge and mylohyoid ridge in particular, careful palpation of the tissues is essential. Prior to impression making, a mental image of the completed denture should be created.

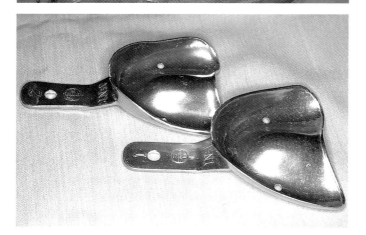

Fig. 9-3　Select stock trays which can cover all the landmarks indicating the denture-bearing area. Since the tray is not evenly spaced from the mucosa and can not be adequately adapted to the shape of the ridge, relatively viscous impression materials must be used.

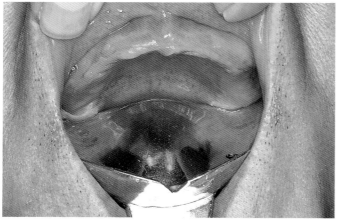

Fig. 9-4　Check the size of the upper impression tray. Position the posterior border of the tray on the hamular notches.

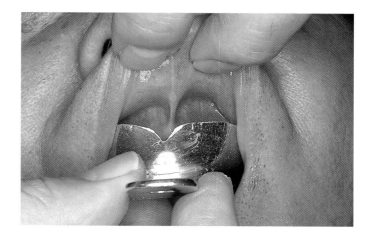

Fig. 9-5 The tray should then be lifted at the front. The borders of the tray should be observed in relation to the anterior ridge. The tray should loosely fit the ridge and have a 3~5 mm space for the impression material.

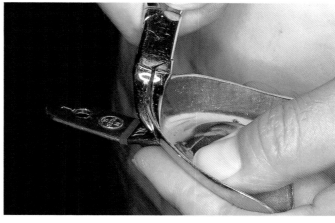

Fig. 9-6 If the gap between the tray and the ridge is too large, especially at the periphery, the impression of the sulcus will be made too wide and indentifying the position of the tissue reflections will be difficult. The tray should be adjusted by bending it beforehand.

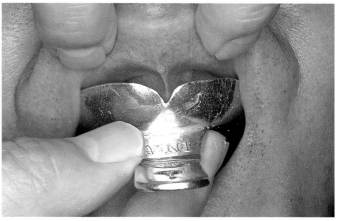

Fig. 9-7 Reduce the border of the tray so that it is somewhat short of the tissue reflection. Adequate clearance is needed in the frenal area.

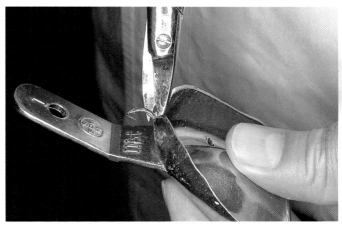

Fig. 9-8 Those areas which are too long can be reduced with scissors. The border must be adequately cleared, particularly in the frenal area.

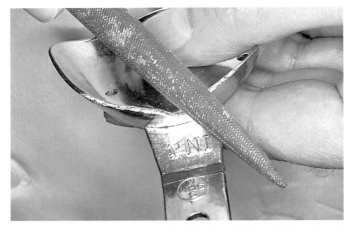

Fig. 9-9 The area which has been cut should be smoothed with a file or carborundum points.

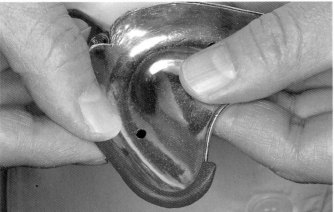

Fig. 9-10 Deficient tray borders are corrected by adding utility wax. Particularly in the buccal space where alginate can not be easily carried, the impression may be underextended because of tray deficiencies.

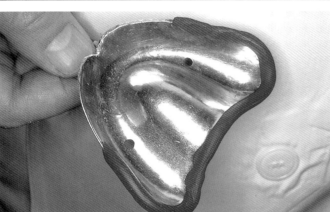

Fig. 9-11 Utility wax is added on the tissue side of the posterior border in order to prevent excess alginate from flowing down the soft palate during impression making.

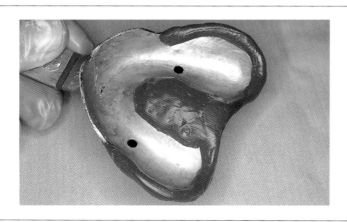

Fig. 1 Displacement of the mucosa may occur in those areas where the tray directly contacts the tissues during the impression procedure. To avoid this, it can be helpful to prepare a stop by adding soft wax on the central portion of the tray. It will also act as a guiding stop to seat the tray in place.

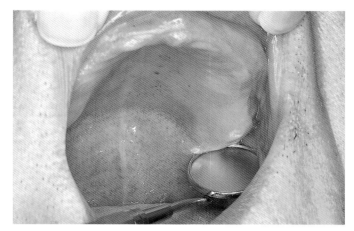

Fig. 9-12 When a mouth mirror is slid posteriorly along the crest of the ridge, its edge drops into a depression, which is the hamular notch. It may be situated more posteriorly than its expected location.

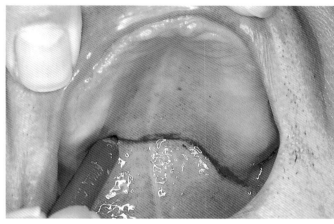

Fig. 9-13 The hamular notches are marked with an indelible pencil. Continuously instruct the patient to say "ah" strongly and mark the vibrating line.

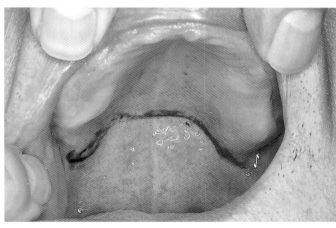

Fig. 9-14 In this patient, the foveae palatinae are indistinct, but usually the vibrating line passes just slightly anterior to the foveae. Therefore, they can be used to determine the posterior border of the maxillary denture.

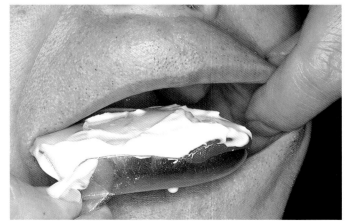

Fig. 9-15 The consistency of the alginate must be thickened by using less water than is usually required. It should be viscous enough so that the alginate can be piled up high on the tray. The tray should be rotated into the mouth with the corner of the mouth retracted using the index finger.

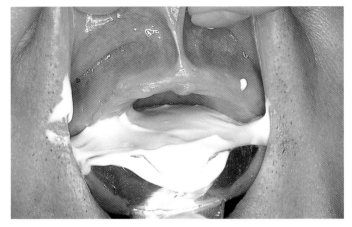

Fig. 9-16 The loaded tray should be seated first at the back of the mouth, and then lifted slowly at the front so that the alginate flows anteriorly. If this procedure is done too quickly, air will be trapped.

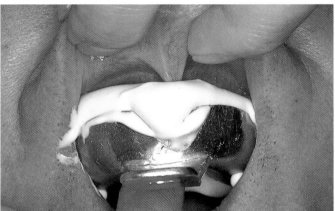

Fig. 9-17 The upper lip should be elevated using the index and middle fingers so that sufficient alginate flows into the labial sulcus. The position of the tray handle should be kept at the midline of the face and used as a centering guide so that the tray can be seated in the correct position.

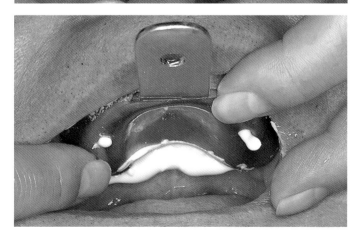

Fig. 9-18 The seating pressure is stopped when the alginate can be observed along the entire posterior border. The tray is still held until the alginate has completely reached the gel state.

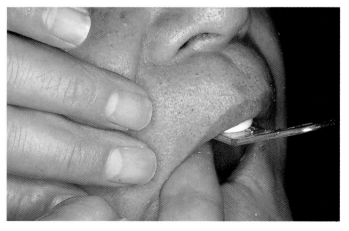

Fig. 9-19 Before gelation has progressed too far, the labial and buccal borders should be molded using finger manipulations.

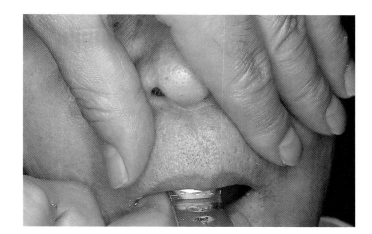

Fig. 9-20   As a thick consistency of alginate is used, border molding should be performed firmly so that the impression is not overextended. The preliminary impression requires that the border be extended, but if the border is extended too far, it will be difficult to identify its position.

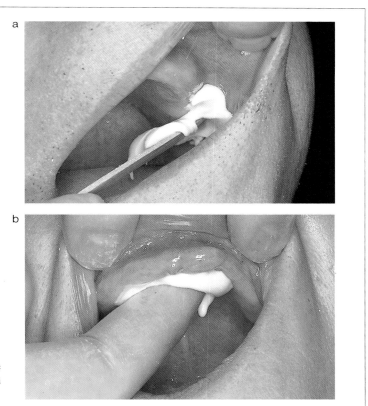

a

b

Fig. 1a, b   Using a spatula or a finger, some alginate should be placed into the vestibule and the deepest area of the palate where the alginate can not be easily carried.

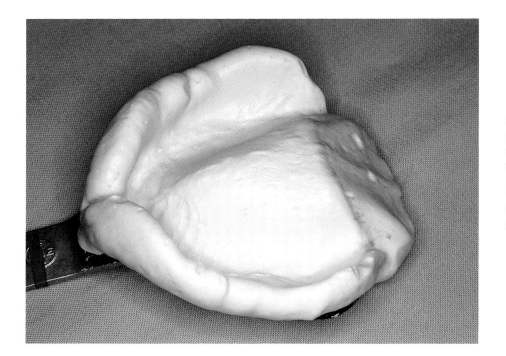

Fig. 9-21 Completed maxillary preliminary impression. It covers all the anatomical landmarks and has round and molded peripheries. The ah-line marked on the palate with an indelible pencil has been transferred onto the surface of the impression.

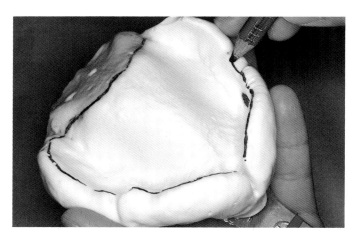

Fig. 9-22 As alginate with a thick consistency is used, the impression tends to be overextended. So the denture outline should be drawn on the impression with an indelible pencil by referring to the anatomical landmarks in the mouth while the patient is still in the chair.

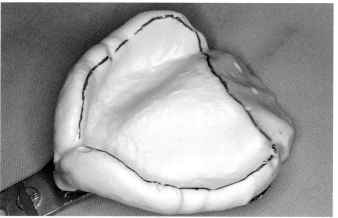

Fig. 9-23 The indelible pencil outline will also be transferred onto the cast and act as a useful guide to the technician when the individual tray is made.

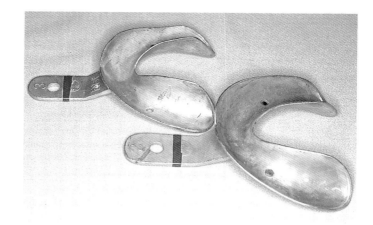

Fig. 9-24 The Britannia metal edentulous tray used for modeling compound is recommended for the alginate. This type of tray can be adjusted to some degree by cutting and bending even for highly resorbed alveolar ridges.

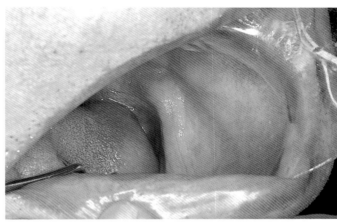

Fig. 9-25 Posteriorly, the retromolar pads should be covered by the tray. The external oblique ridge and mylohyoid ridge should be recognized not only by observation but also by careful palpation.

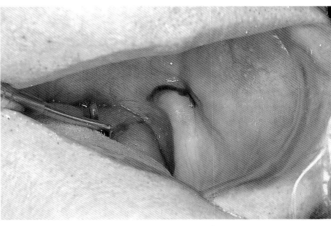

Fig. 9-26 In cases where the retromolar pad is indistinct, it should be marked with an indelible pencil prior to making the impression.

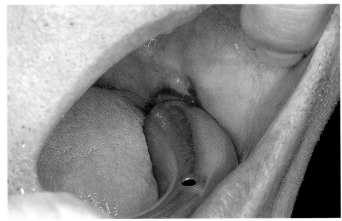

Fig. 9-27 Observe the posterior extension of the tray in relation to the retromolar pad when positioning the tray over the anterior alveolar ridge. Buccally, the tray should be resting against the external oblique ridge.

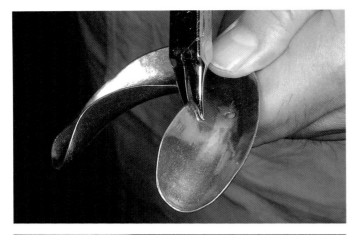

Fig. 9-28   In cases with a severely resorbed ridge, it is difficult to fit the stock tray adequately to its complicated contour. The tray should be roughly adjusted by bending and then a viscous impression material must be used to cover the deficiencies.

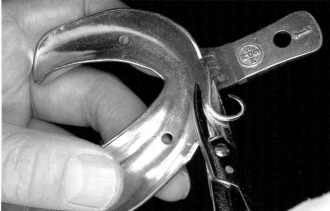

Fig. 9-29   A border that is too long should be cut with scissors. If the tray border is too long, the impression will be grossly overextended and too wide, making it impossible to identify the position of the tissue reflection. The roughened edge should be smoothed with a file.

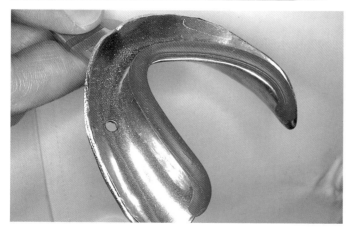

Fig. 9-30   Any deficient tray border can be corrected by adding utility wax. The wax is also used on the entire lingual border to easily carry the alginate into the lingual sulcus. Not using utility wax, will result in knife-edged and irregular borders.

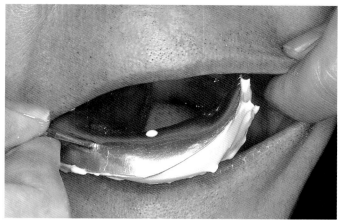

Fig. 9-31 Especially in cases with a severely resorbed ridge, the alginate is mixed using much less water than is used for the maxilla. Alginate with a thick consistency can push the surrounding soft tissues away and capture the total anatomical form of the alveolar ridge. The patient is asked to raise the tongue slightly and the tray is rotated into the mouth.

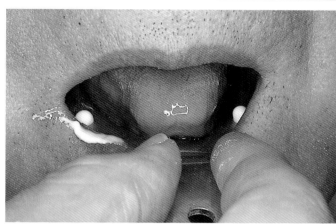

Fig. 9-32 Ensure that the tray handle is positioned at the midline of the face. Before gelation of the alginate has progressed too far, the patient should be asked to protrude the tip of the tongue and move it from side to side. These actions help push the alginate which has collected lingually out of the lingual sulcus and mold an appropriate lingual border.

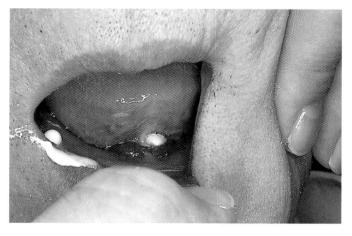

Fig. 9-33 The fingers are used to gently mold the labial and buccal areas, producing round and molded borders. As these consecutive procedures are time-consuming for a beginner, it is recommended to use iced water for delaying gelation of the alginate.

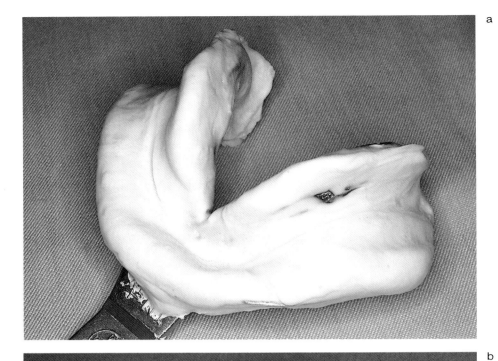

a

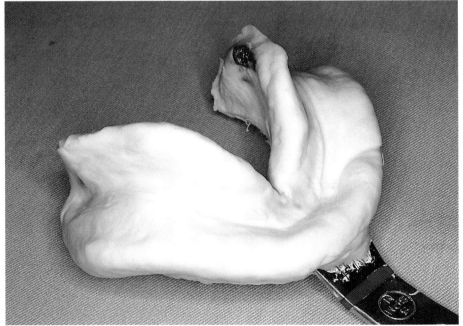

b

Fig. 9-34a, b Check whether or not the completed impression contains all the denture-bearing area by referring to the anatomical landmarks such as the external oblique ridge, mylohyoid ridge and retromolar pad. The preliminary impression should extend beyond the limits of the final impression so that an individual tray can be made from it. Even though small air bubbles are present on the impression surface, some of the utility wax borders appear to be elevated away from the surface or the tray has exposed areas, if they are not very severe, they can be overlooked because they can be corrected on the preliminary cast.

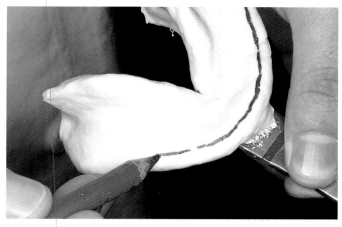

Fig. 9-35 The denture outline should be marked with an indelible pencil on the impression surface by referring to the anatomical landmarks in the mouth. This procedure is essential for providing information about the denture-bearing area for the technician who has not seen the patient's mouth. Without this information, the individual tray can not be made.

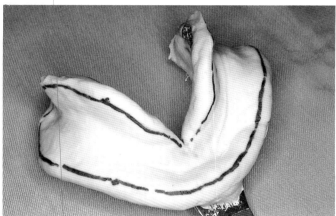

Fig. 9-36 The estimated denture outline is marked on the areas corresponding to the external oblique ridge, 4 to 5 mm below the mylohyoid ridge, a point on the retromolar pad 2/3 of the way from the anterior border, and mucolabial, mucobuccal and mucolingual reflections.

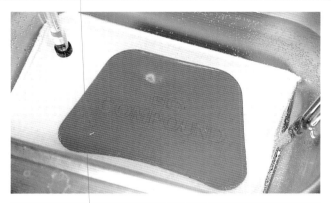

Fig. 1 In cases with severe bone resorption, it is difficult to fit the stock tray to the ridge and sometimes it is even impossible. As there is a limit to increasing the viscosity of the alginate, its use must be abandoned. The following procedure will be somewhat complicated, but the fit of the tray can be improved by using a layer of modeling compound between the tray and alginate.

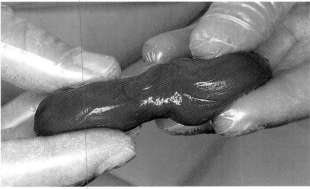

Fig. 2 Modeling compound softened in a water bath should be kneaded and rolled into a cylinder-shaped form.

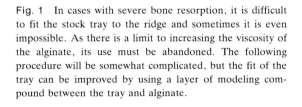

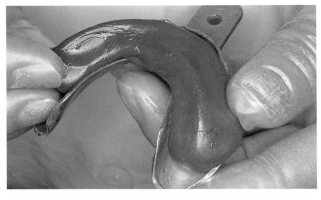

Fig. 3 The compound should be placed in the tray, which has been roughly adjusted according to the form of the mandibular ridge. It should be spread in excess in the molar regions.

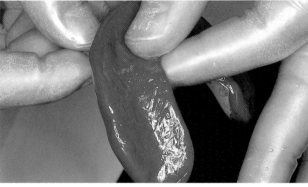

Fig. 4 The compound should be molded with the fingers by referring to the ridge form.

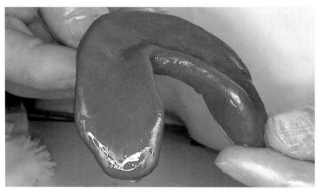

Fig. 5 It should be extended beyond the mylohyoid ridge lingually and about as far as the external oblique ridge buccally.

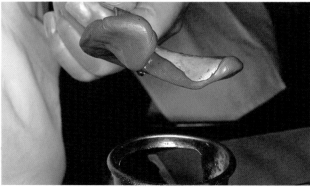

Fig. 6 The compound should be gently warmed above a flame so as to ensure that the entire surface is softened.

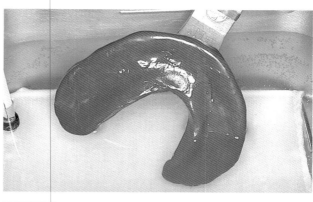

Fig. 7   Before inserting the tray into the mouth, the compound should be tempered in a warm water bath.

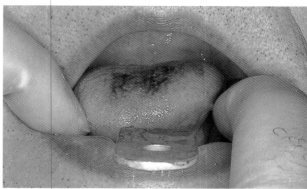

Fig. 8   The patient is asked to raise the tongue slightly and the tray is rotated into the mouth with the corner of the mouth retracted by a finger. Keeping the position of the tray handle at the midline of the face, the tray should be gently seated.

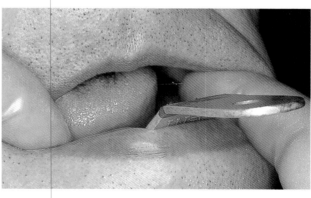

Fig. 9   The tray should be seated into position by pressure from the index fingers on the tray with the mandible supported by the thumbs and held steadily in place. The patient is instructed to move the tongue in order to actively push the compound which has collected lingually out of the sulcus. Also the patient should be asked to purse the lips or finger manipulations should be used to mold the labial and buccal borders so that they will not be over extended.

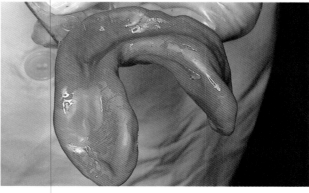

Fig. 10   It is essential that the impression should cover all the denture-bearing area. If creases are present, they can be disregarded because this impression will be converted into a tray.

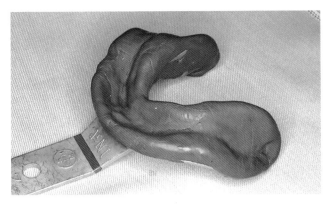

Fig. 11 If any short areas are noted after observing all the vestibules, more compound should be added in these areas and partially remolded.

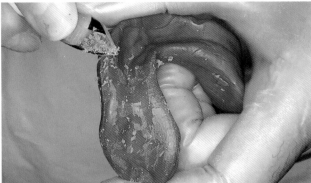

Fig. 12 By referring to the anatomical landmarks, over-extensions should be trimmed with a knife. Then all the borders should be reduced by about 2-3 mm.

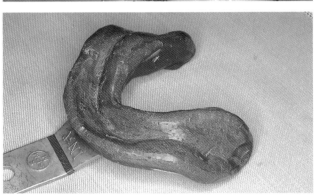

Fig. 13 The entire inside of the modeling compound impression should be scraped away to a depth of 1-2 mm in order to create a space for the alginate impression material. The compound impression has now been converted into a tray with an improved fit.

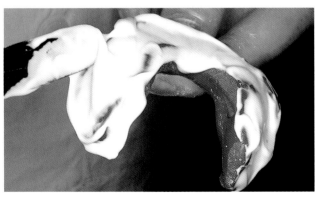

Fig. 14 Alginate mixed using more water than usual should be evenly spread over the entire inside surface of the compound tray. It should be inserted using a similar technique to that used in the usual alginate impression.

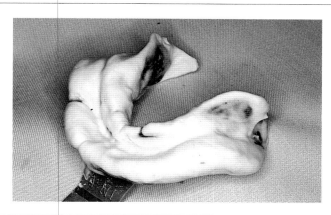

Fig. 15 The completed preliminary impression made with alginate using a compound tray. As an alginate adhesive is not used, care must be taken not to use too much pressure upon removal. The lips and cheeks should be reflected so that the borders are fully exposed to break the seal, so the impression can be easily removed without separation between the alginate and modeling compound.

a

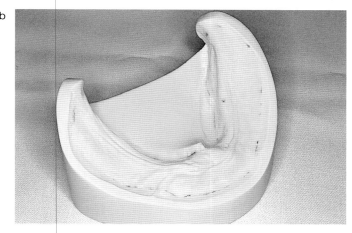

b

Fig. 9-37a, b Completed maxillary and mandibular preliminary casts. The indelible pencil outline has been transferred onto the cast. It will serve as a useful guide when the individual tray is made. All the land areas should be trimmed low in order to facilitate fabrication of the custom tray.

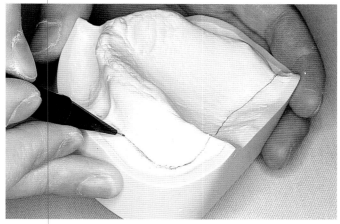

Fig. 9-38 The denture outline is accentuated with a pencil. The outline for the custom tray should be then drawn 2-3 mm short of the denture outline.

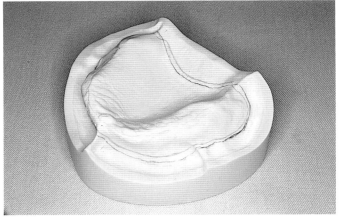

Fig. 9-39 The posterior border of the tray should be marked 2-3 mm distal to the estimated denture border. Extending the impression somewhat distal to the posterior border of the denture will provide a guiding surface when carving the post-dam on the cast.

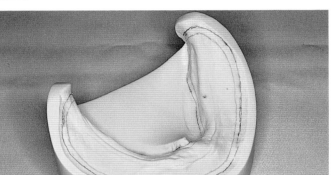

Fig. 9-40 Also on the mandibular cast, the denture outline is accentuated and then the tray outline is marked 2-3 mm short of the denture outline. As the estimated denture outline has been given, it is easy to determine the outline for the custom tray.

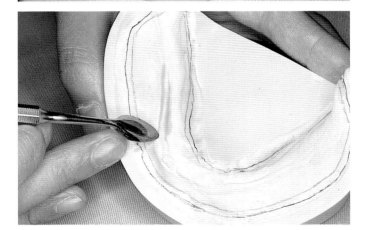

Fig. 9-41 Baseplate wax should be added to provide relief over tori, sharp edges, and flabby areas. Then the undercuts of the anterior labial and posterior lingual regions should be blocked out with wax.

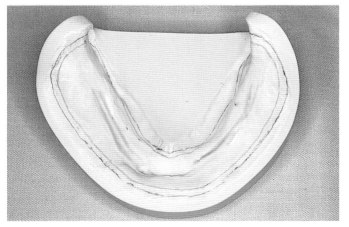

Fig. 9-42 Generally, a layer of baseplate wax is added onto the cast to provide a relief space for the tray. It is performed to minimize the displacement of the soft tissues covering the palate and residual ridges when making the final impression. However, if excessive pressure is not used when seating the tray, this kind of relief is not necessary. There will be greater dimensional changes during polymerization of the denture than the deformation that takes place when the tissue is displaced while making the impression without a spacer. When considering this, it is not worth using a spacer. The inner surface of the denture corresponding to the displacement can be adjusted by using pressure-indicating paste at the time of denture insertion.

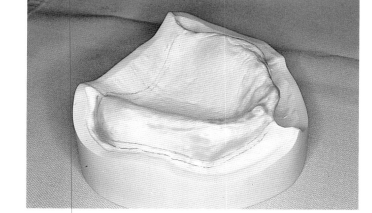

Fig. 9-43 Wax is added to provide relief over the rugae, incisive papilla, torus palatinus and flabby areas. Any undercuts should also be blocked out.

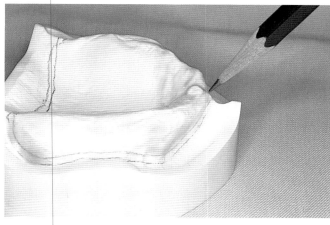

Fig. 9-44 The anterior region of the maxilla tends to be excessively blocked out. When considering undercuts which may need blocking out, the cast should be viewed from the path of insertion and removal of the tray, not from directly above the cast. The angle between this direction and the occlusal plane is about 45 degrees.

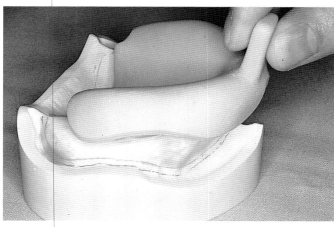

Fig. 9-45 Anteriorly, excessive blocking out will place the tray border away from the ridge leading to faulty border molding or an excessively thick border.

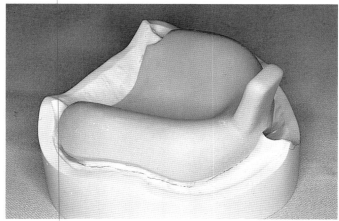

Fig. 9-46 The handle should be positioned in approximately the same position as the anterior teeth were, with a similar inclination to that of the teeth so that it will not distort the lip during border molding. Also, the top of the handle should not be bent. Otherwise it will interfere with the normal position of the lip.

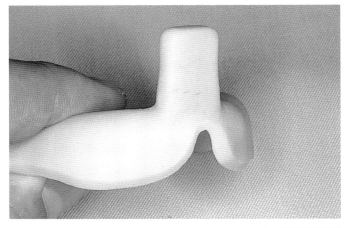

Fig. 9-47 In order to easily add compound to the border and also provide strong adhesion between the tray and compound, the tray border should be beveled so that the area coming into contact with the compound increases.

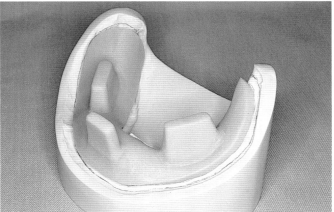

Fig. 9-48 Finger rests should be made bilaterally in the first molar region of the lower individual tray. The lower tray should be made somewhat thicker than the upper tray. In the case with a flat ridge, the portion between the handle and finger rest should be reinforced by placing extra tray material on the area between them.

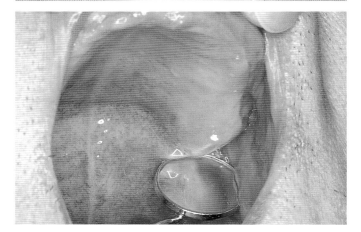

Fig. 9-49 When a mouth mirror is slid posteriorly along the crest of the residual ridge, its edge drops into a displaceable depression, the hamular notch. The posterior border should be placed in this region. By using this cushion the peripheral seal can be established.

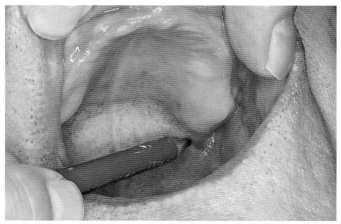

Fig. 9-50 If the posterior border is situated on the maxillary tuberosity, a peripheral seal can not be expected from this nonresilient tissue. Most poorly retentive dentures may be inadequately extended here. The notch should be marked with an indelible pencil.

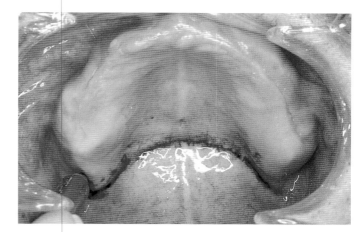

Fig. 9-51 The distal end of the upper denture should be placed on the vibrating line(ah-line). The line can be recognized as a fold when asking the patient to say "ah" and relax. It should be marked with an indelible pencil.

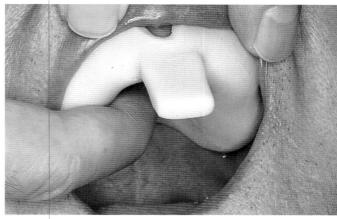

Fig. 9-52 When the tray is inserted, the ah-line marked with an indelible pencil will be transferred onto the fitting surface of the tray. It will indicate how much to trim the posterior border. As the posterior border of the tray has been determined according to the ah-line on the preliminary cast, which was transferred from the preliminary impression, gross corrections will not be required.

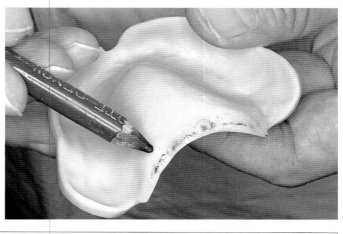

Fig. 9-53 Overextensions are easily trimmed with a carbide bur, but the correction of underextensions is more complicated. A deficient border should be extended appropriately on the preliminary cast with self-curing resin. The compound should not be used for extension. When additional compound is added on the tissue side of the posterior border of the tray and pressure is applied to the mucosa(Fig 9- 77, 78), the extended compound border of the tray will be somewhat softened and can not support the additional compound firmly.

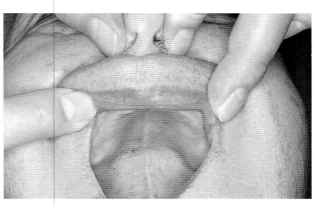

Fig. 1 The ah-line can be located by blowing out through the nose with closed nostrils so that the soft palate expands downwards. This method may be useful in cases where the boundary line of motion in the soft palate generated by the "ah" sound is not obvious.

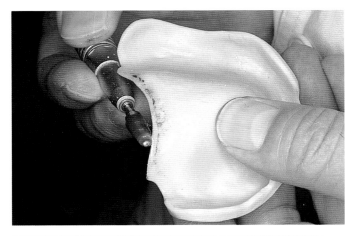

Fig. 9-54   The posterior border of the tray should be trimmed to about 2 mm beyond the vibrating line.

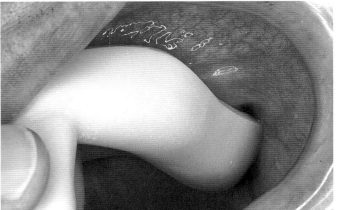

Fig. 9-55   Other areas should be checked by observation to ensure the tray has the correct extension. The tray should be some 2 mm short of the base of the sulcus as seen with the cheek lifted by the fingers. This tray has the correct extension in the buccal space, but it is overextended in the buccal frenal area.

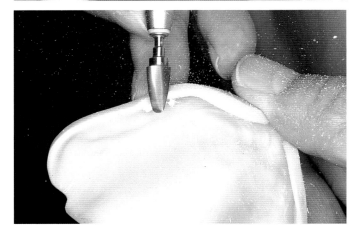

Fig. 9-56   The tray should be reduced with a carbide bur until it has the correct extension. The areas necessary for correction should be marked with a pencil in the mouth so that mistakes will not be made when trimming.

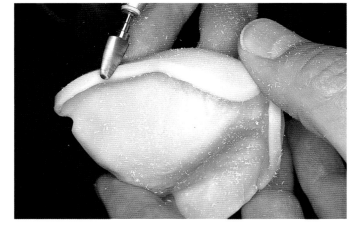

Fig. 9-57   The reduced borders should again be beveled so that compound can be easily added(cf. Fig 9-47). Also the internal surface of the border should be slightly beveled. As a result, the border will be covered with compound on the inside and outside when it is added to the tray, thus firmly adhering to the tray.

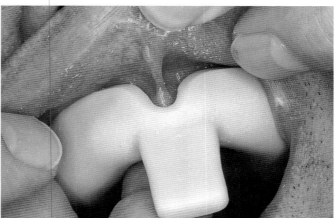

Fig. 9-58   Correctly extended impression tray. The border tends to be overtrimmed for fear of movement of the reflection area. If underextended, it will be difficult to handle the compound because due to its increased width, it loses support.

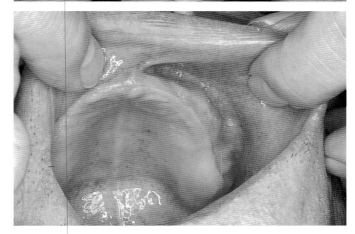

Fig. 9-59   Extra clearance should be provided for the frenal areas. Especially for the buccal frenum, wider clearance is needed due to its horizontal and of course vertical movement.

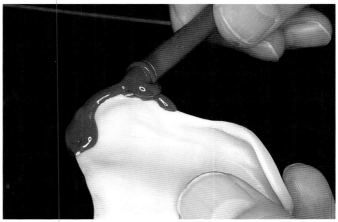

Fig. 9-60   The length of the denture border will be adequate if the sulcus is recorded as deeply as it is observed. When the lip and cheek are pulled in an exaggerated fashion to mimic the functional situation, the border is liable to be underextended. Using this action, it is difficult to determine the direction and amount of force used in actual functional movements.

Fig. 9-61   The periphery of the tray should be border molded in 5-6 sections. First, the softened compound (Red compound, KERR) should be added on the tray border from the hamular notch to the buccal space.

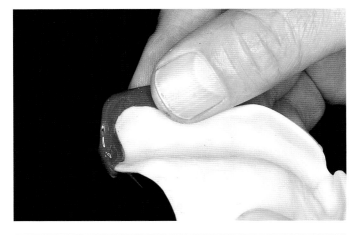

Fig. 9-62   The added compound should be molded so as to mimick the shape of the final border by pinching the compound with the fingers. Any irregularities should be also corrected. The buccal space should be closely observed. If it is broad, an appropriate amount of compound should be added as needed.

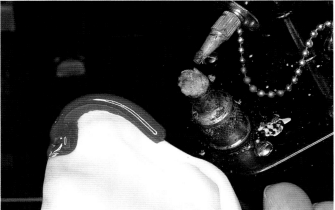

Fig. 9-63   The compound gradually stiffens during this process, so it should be softened again with an alcohol torch, taking care not to burn it. If the compound is boiled or ignited, it will lose its flow characteristics because important constituents will have evaporated.

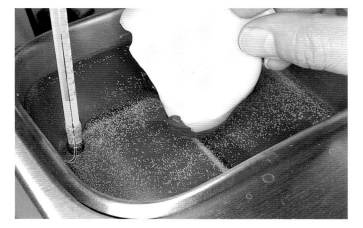

Fig. 9-64   As the softened compound can scald the mucosa, it should be tempered in a warm water bath before the tray is inserted into the mouth.

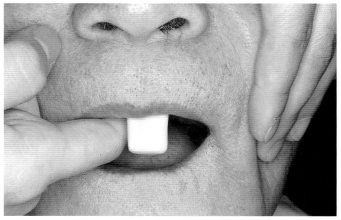

Fig. 9-65   The tray should be rotated into the mouth so that the softened compound will not be deformed by the lips. The tray should be firmly held with the finger and the cheek should be gently massaged with the hand so that the sulcus will be recorded just as it is seen.

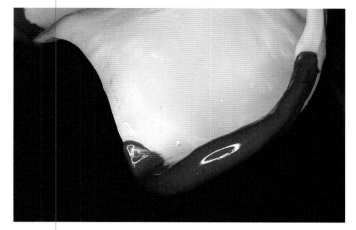

Fig. 9-66   If the softened compound is stiff when the tray is inserted into the mouth or the material added on the border is insufficient and does not come into contact with the tissues adequately, the compound will have a shiny surface.

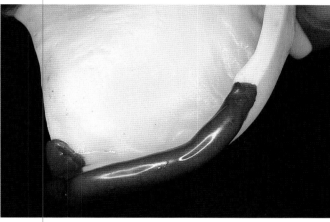

Fig. 9-67   If the compound is appropriately molded with the tissues, it will have a mat surface. The molded border should be checked to ensure that the hamular notch and buccal space are appropriately recorded by referring to them in the mouth. In cases with a thickly molded border in the buccal space, its width should be checked using the technique described previously(p. 36).

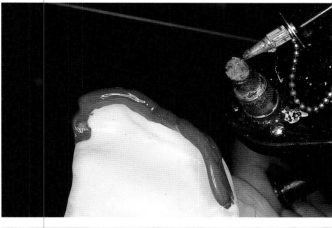

Fig. 9-68   The border molding should be continued in the adjacent buccal frenal area, or on the posterior buccal border of the opposite side. For the buccal frenal area, the buccal sulcus should be recorded first, when the cheek is relaxed. The compound around the notch for the buccal frenum should then be softened again with an alcohol torch and tempered before insertion of the tray.

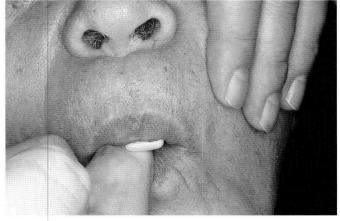

Fig. 9-69   As the movements of the buccal frenum are horizontal as well as vertical, wider clearance is needed around the buccal frenum. Generally, the frenum runs obliquely and posteriorly, therefore it should be recorded with its anterior movement by pursing the lips such as when whistling, during border molding. A V-shaped notch will then be obtained.

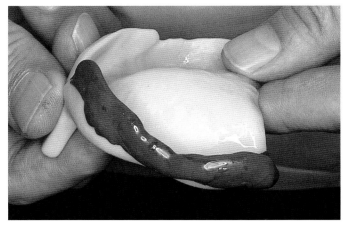

Fig. 9-70 The functional record of the buccal frenum that hardly appeared on the preliminary impression has been recorded in the compound. This molded buccal border has a wide notch for the buccal frenum.

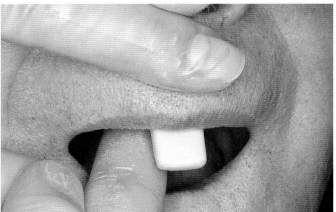

Fig. 9-71 As the compound does not easily flow out anteriorly, the lip should be massaged with the fingers so as to push the excess material out of the sulcus. After removal, the molded border should be examined by referring to the sulcus, and if too thick, should be adjusted with a sharp knife.

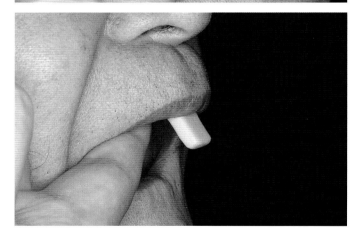

Fig. 9-72 When the border is molded, the upper lip looks too prominent because the lower lip is unsupported. So, generally, the labial border is liable to be molded too thin. The thickness of the lost tissues should be estimated using the incisive papilla as a guide and then the thickness of the border determined.

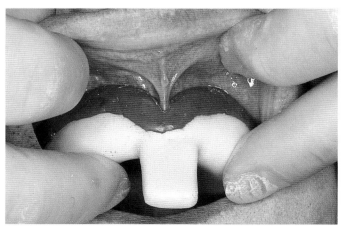

Fig. 9-73 Due to compound's poor flow properties, sometimes the impression of the frenum may not be clearly recorded. In such a case, firstly the notch should be widened and deepened with a sharp knife by referring to the frenum.

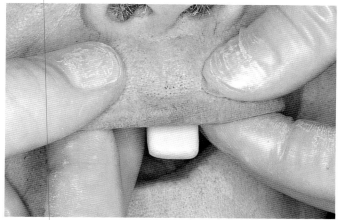

Fig. 9-74   Only the compound around the notch should be gently softened using an alcohol torch with a pin-point flame. The upper lip should be actively manipulated in a vertical direction. Even if forcefully manipulated, portions of the border other than the notch that were not softened will not be reduced.

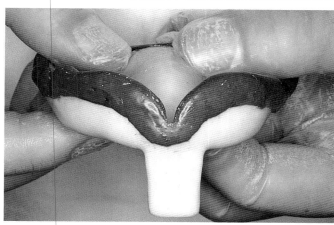

Fig. 9-75   As the action of the lip in this area is mainly vertical, manipulation in a horizontal direction that causes lateral movement of the frenum should not be performed. A labial notch that is too wide could lead to a loss of seal, especially in patients with a short and active lip.

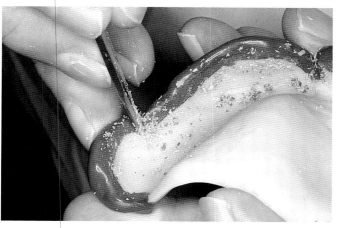

Fig. 9-76   The excess compound that flowed on the tissue side of the tray should be trimmed off with a knife. If it remains, the soft tissue contour will be distorted with the compound extending from the impression surface of the final impression material.

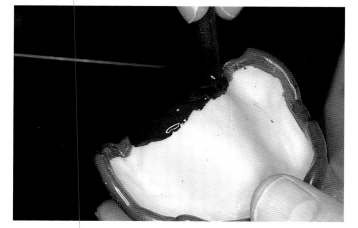

Fig. 9-77   Compound with good flow properties(Green compound, KERR) should be placed on the fitting surface of the tray along the posterior border to produce displacement of the soft tissues in the posterior seal area.

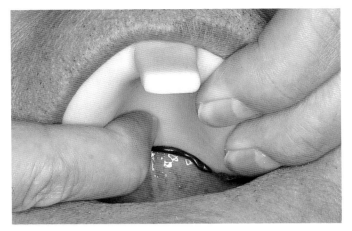

Fig. 9-78 After the added compound is softened again, the tray should be seated in the mouth and firm pressure applied toward the palate with a finger. The tray should be held in place under load for a while. The compound will be pressed into the soft mucosa leading to a better peripheral seal.

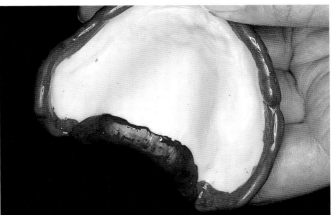

Fig. 9-79 The posterior palatal seal has been completed, so if the patient is asked to widely open the mouth or the tray is pulled down, the tray will not be displaced. When the retention is poor, there is probably a leak in the seal. It should be located and corrected. Usually it is due to a leak in the hamular notch region. Also an inadequate buccal border in the buccal space may cause poor retention.

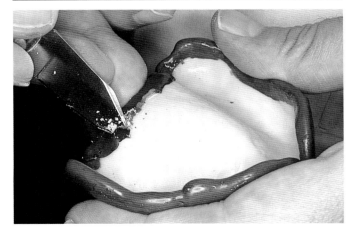

Fig. 9-80 Compound on the fitting surface of the posterior border should be tapered with a knife to form a smooth surface between the compound and the tray.

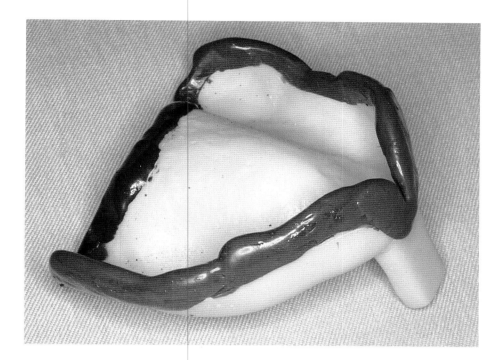

Fig. 9-81　The border-molded maxillary custom tray. The final impression should not be performed until the tray has good retention.

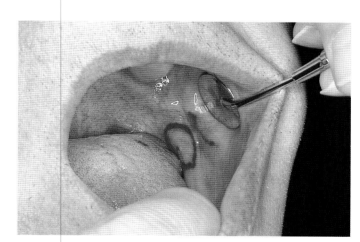

Fig. 9-82　The tray borders should be examined in turn by referring to the anatomical landmarks for impression making and corrections should be made as needed. The outline of the retromolar pad should be marked with an indelible pencil. In some cases it is indistinct, but in most cases its contour can be grasped by careful observation and palpation.

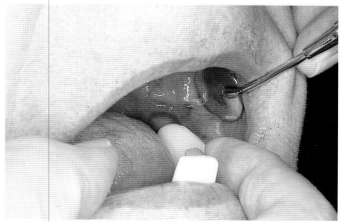

Fig. 9-83　As the posterior peripheral seal can be obtained by placing the denture border over the resilient glandular tissue, the posterior half of the retromolar pad, the denture must cover more than half of the pad. Therefore, the posterior border of the tray should be corrected so that it covers the anterior half of the pad.

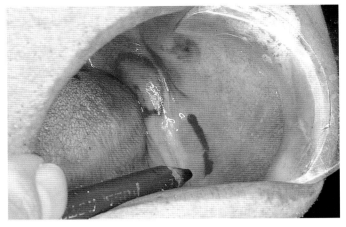

Fig. 9-84 The bony ridge that runs anteroposteriorly outside the buccal shelf can be found by palpation. Beginners will find it useful to mark the ridge with an indelible pencil.

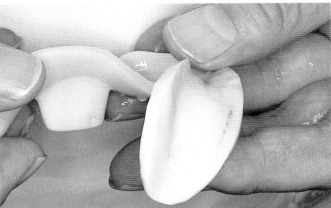

Fig. 9-85 The pencil mark is transferred to the fitting surface of the tray when it is seated in the mouth.

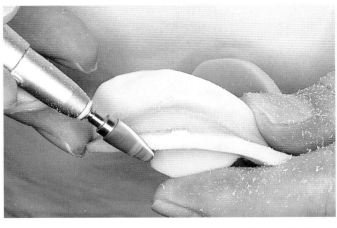

Fig. 9-86 The denture border can be extended 1-2 mm beyond the external oblique ridge, so the tray border should be resting against the ridge. The recording of details in the peripheral area will be left to the compound during border molding.

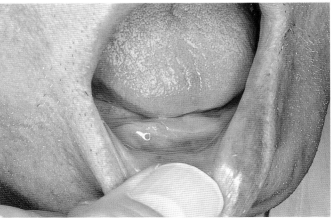

Fig. 9-87 When the patient is instructed to close the mouth slightly with relaxed lips and the lower lip is pulled lightly outwards, the depth of the sulcus which is seen should be used as a guide for determining the denture border.

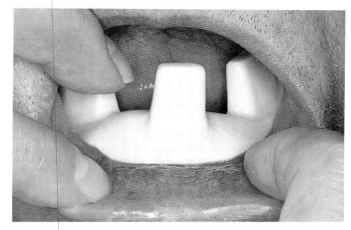

Fig. 9-88 This tray is somewhat overextended.

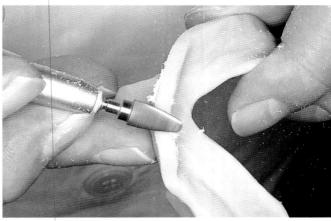

Fig. 9-89 The tray should be reduced. This process may make the border of the tray thicker. It must be corrected by observing the depth and width of the sulcus and tapering the border.

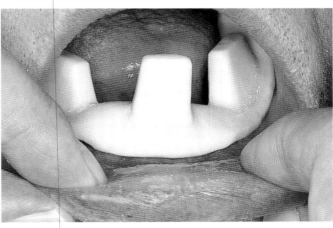

Fig. 9-90 The tray should be inserted again into the mouth and evaluated by manipulating the lip as described in Fig. 9-87. If the lip is pulled too vigorously, the sulcus will become too shallow because the mental muscle attachment is situated high.

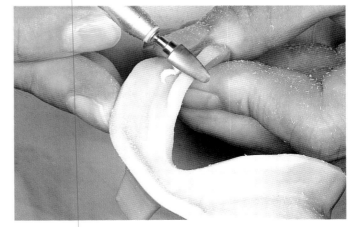

Fig. 9-91 When alginate has been used for the preliminary impression, the lingual border of the tray requires few corrections. After observation and palpation it should, if necessary, be corrected.

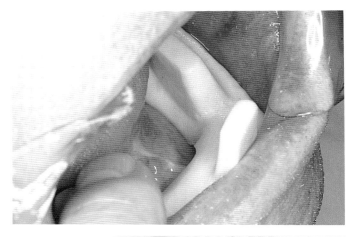

Fig. 9-92 The border of this tray comes in contact with the floor of the mouth in the sublingual gland area. It is somewhat overextended.

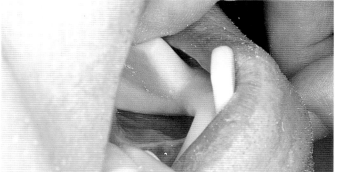

Fig. 9-93 Clearance should be provided between the tray border and the mucosa of the floor of the mouth, and recording of its fine relationship with the mucosa will be left to the compound.

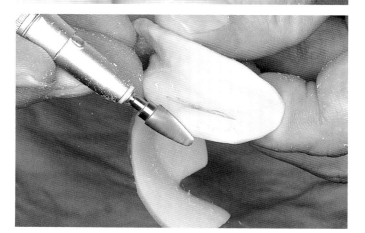

Fig. 9-94 The bony ridge should be found by palpation in the mylohyoid ridge area, and the tray border should be trimmed slightly beyond the ridge.

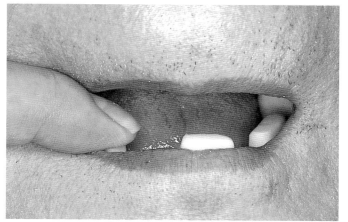

Fig. 9-95 When the tray is appropriately adjusted, it will not be raised in the mouth and will remain in place. If it is pushed with a finger, it will not be easily displaced.

Fig. 9-96   The posterior peripheral seal can be obtained by placing the posterior border on the posterior half of the retromolar pad which is made up of resilient glandular tissues. The border can be located anywhere on the glandular tissue, but if the denture border is placed too far posteriorly, some patients will complain of tightness at the base of the tongue. So, the distal end should be placed at a point 2/3 of the way up the retromolar pad.

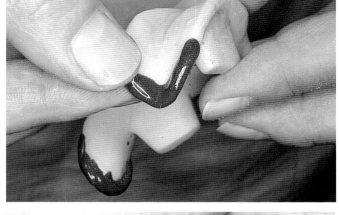

Fig. 9-97   The added compound should be softened with an alcohol torch and tempered. The tray should be reinserted into the mouth and gently seated in place. The compound should not be added directly onto the tray resin. If the compound is supported in this fashion, excess pressure will be applied onto the pad during border molding leading to gross deformation of the pad.

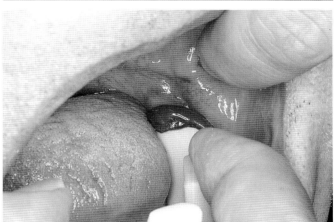

Fig. 9-98   The compound should be added continuously on the buccal border anterior to the retromolar pad. It should be extended somewhat beyond the external oblique ridge while its irregularities are corrected with the fingers.

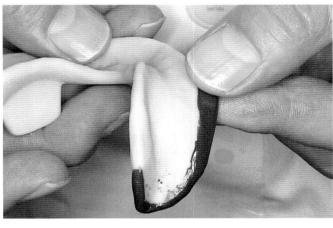

Fig. 9-99   The tray should be inserted into the mouth and seated in place. The softened compound should be actively pushed into the sulcus with the index finger of the free hand. This process should be repeated until the border is adequately extended and the external oblique ridge is recorded on the compound.

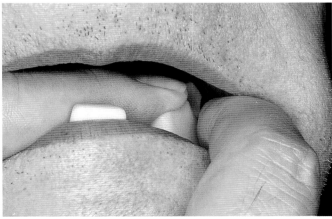

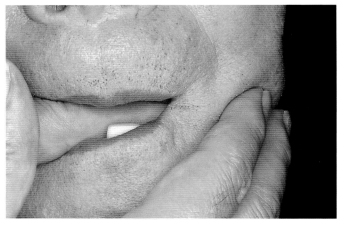

Fig. 9-100 After the border has been adequately extended, it should be built up by adding extra compound. The surface of the compound should be slightly softened, the tray reseated, and the cheek gently massaged in the area corresponding to the external oblique ridge.

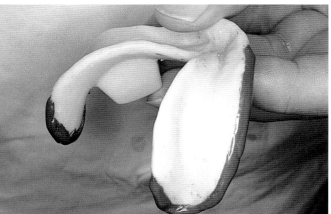

Fig. 9-101 The border should be smooth, round, and convex, conforming well to the contour of the buccal pouch. In cases with a concave ridge, the external oblique ridge can not even be guessed, so its concavity should be recorded just as it is.

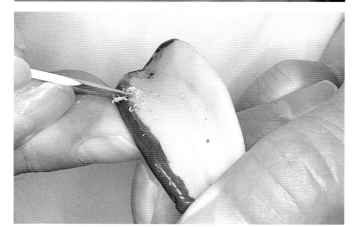

Fig. 9-102 Excess compound that flowed onto the fitting surface of the tray should be removed with a sharp knife to form a smooth surface between the compound and the tray.

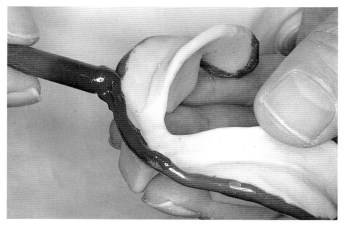

Fig. 9-103 Then the labial and buccal borders should be molded. In the frenal areas, border molding should be actively performed using a similar technique to that used in the upper jaw. A wide notch has been molded for the right buccal frenum.

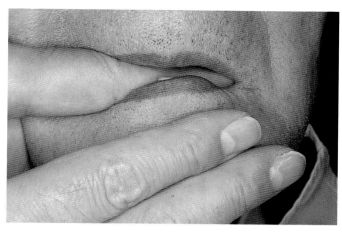

Fig. 9-104 Finger manipulations and lip movements by the patient should not be used to mold the labial border. Excessive movements may be the cause of underextended borders leading to a decrease in the peripheral seal. By gently massaging the lower lip, the depth of the vestibule with a relaxed lip should be recorded in the compound just as it is.

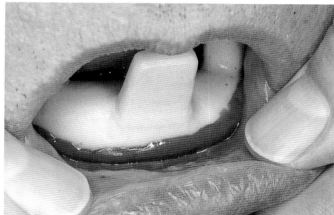

Fig. 9-105 When the lower lip is lightly pulled outwards, the length of the molded compound border should conform to the depth of the labial vestibule. In patients with strong muscle tension in this region, the impression border is liable to become too thin and too short. So the contour of the border should be appropriately contoured by observing the width and depth of the vestibule with a relaxed lip. But actually, in such a case, the border should be molded somewhat thinner than the width of the observed vestibule.

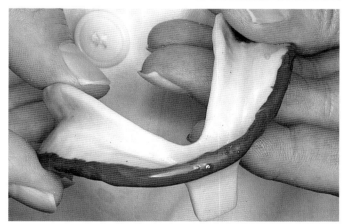

Fig. 9-106 In this way, a portion of the mentalis muscle will be covered by the denture base. So the impression surface of the completed denture should be carefully adjusted using pressure-indicating paste. In this case, the inferior labial frenum is indistinct, but it need not be recorded by forcefully pulling the lower lip outwards.

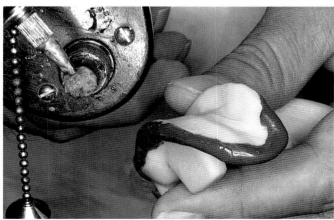

Fig. 9-107 On the buccal side of the retromolar pad, the border is influenced by the action of the masseter muscle. When the masseter muscle contracts, its enlargement indirectly presses the denture border through the cramped buccinator muscle. Therefore if the action of the masseter muscle in function is not recorded, the mucosa in this region will be pressed against the posterior buccal border of the denture during mastication. So, the compound that has been molded in this area should be softened again with an alcohol torch.

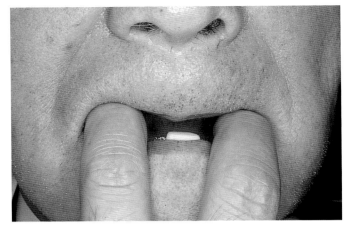

Fig. 9-108 The tray should be reinserted into the mouth and forcefully seated in place. The movement of the masseter muscle is recorded in the compound border by creating its reactive contraction through exertion of a downward pressure on the tray using the fingers.

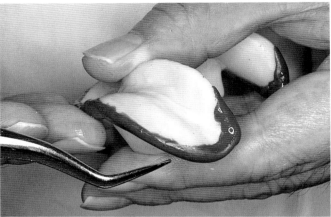

Fig. 9-109 The effect of the masseter muscle has been registered on the distobuccal border. Active contraction creates a concavity and less active contraction leads to a convex border.

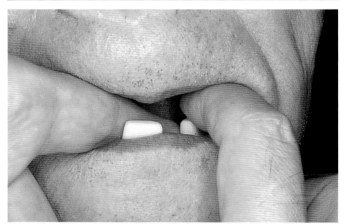

Fig. 9-110 The lingual border is then molded. In most cases, the posterior border should not be lengthened into the retromylohyoid fossa(cf. p. 27). In the mylohyoid ridge area, no tongue movement should be performed during impression making. The patient should be asked only to relax the tongue comfortably and the impression should be made 4-6 mm below the mylohyoid ridge. The tray should be seated in place and the compound on the border should be actively extended beyond the mylohyoid ridge with the index finger of the free hand. In cases of a high membranous attachment on the floor of the mouth, the borders tend to be mistakenly shortened because the dentist may be deceived by this appearance.

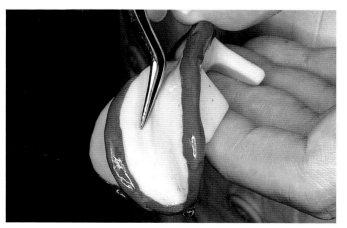

Fig. 9-111 The length of the portion extended beyond the mylohyoid ridge should be checked. If the custom tray is underextended and the length of the compound is increased, the compound tends to be too thin due to the pressure of the tongue. The thin border should be reinforced with extra compound from the outside, or distortion will occur upon removal of the tray.

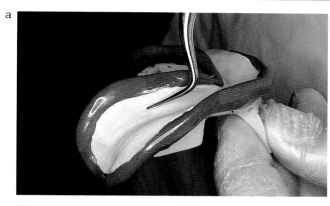

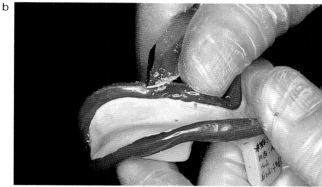

Fig. 1a, b Even in cases when it is favorable to further extend the border inferiorly, the border should be trimmed approximately 5 mm below the mylohyoid ridge. Denture retention and stability may be a little better with the lengthened border, but some patients complain of tightness at the base of the tongue in lengthened cases. So the border should be extended only as far as necessary.

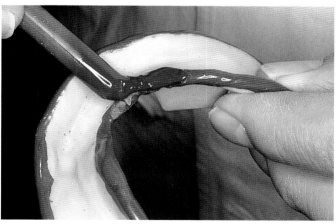

Fig. 9-112 Compound is applied to the border in the sublingual gland area. In this area, exaggerated tongue movements in border molding may be the cause of an underextended denture periphery.

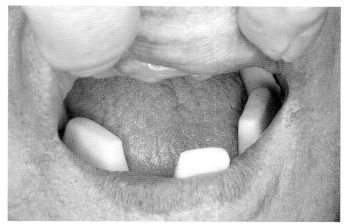

Fig. 9-113 The patient should never be instructed to perform any movements of the tongue, but asked only to relax the tongue comfortably. The depth of the lingual vestibule should be recorded in this situation, that is, the "impression position" of the tongue(cf. P. 28). This will be used as the length of the lingual flange in this area.

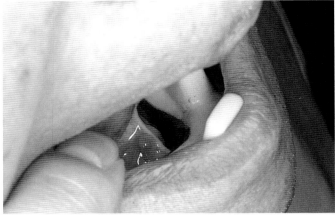

Fig. 9-114 When the space between the tray border and the floor of the mouth is filled with compound, the peripheral seal is completed. Compound should be added onto the border until it comes in contact with the mucosa on the floor of the mouth.

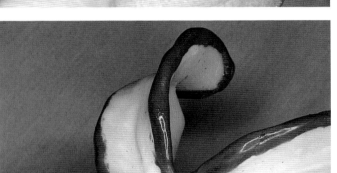

Fig. 9-115 At the genial tubercles, the border should be extended over the tubercles. However, as the genioglossus muscle and the overlying lingual frenum actively move, these movements should be recorded exactly during border molding. This is the only area where the functional movement of the tongue is necessary during impression making. Only the compound in this area should be softened and the patient asked to make some overactive tongue movement such as protrusion.

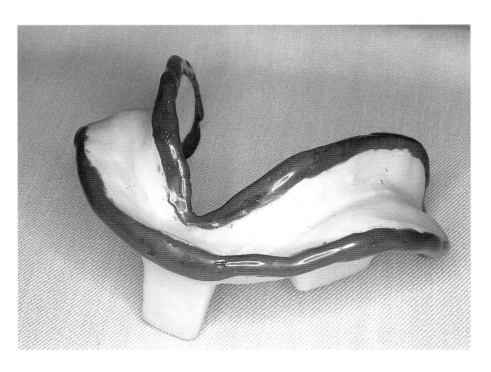

Fig. 9-116 The border-molded mandibular tray. The borders should be smooth and rounded because there are no unnaturally pointed areas in the mouth. The notches for the frena are definite and adequate clearance is provided for the lingual frenum. If lingual border molding is performed appropriately, a point of directional change will occur on the compound border between the mylohyoid area and sublingual area. Therefore, the presence of this point is a good indicator to judge the quality of lingual border molding.

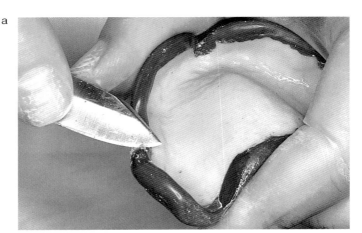

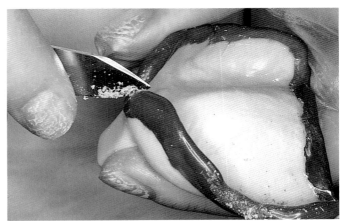

Fig. 9-117a, b   The molded compound borders should be partially corrected prior to making the final impression. If there are any irregularities in the smoothness of the border, they should be trimmed smoothly with a sharp knife. It is left to the final impression material to record the details of the impression in the frenal areas, Therefore a much wider clearance should be provided for the notch.

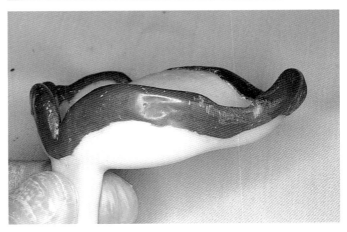

Fig. 9-118   Wider clearance should be provided by increasing the width of the notch for the labial frenum and expanding the size of the V-shaped notch for the buccal frenum.

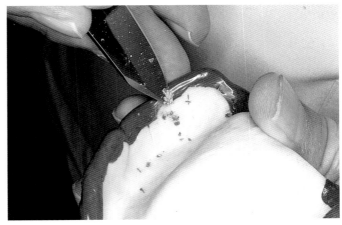

Fig. 9-119   The tissue side of the tray should be carefully examined again. If excess compound has flowed onto the tray, the compound should be trimmed smooth, or it will compress the mucosa when making the final impression.

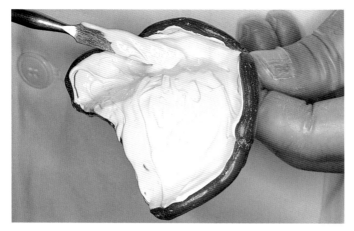

Fig. 9-120 Zinc oxide-eugenol paste, being free-flowing, should be used for the final impression. If a rubber base impression material which has a poor flow is used, the border will be widely extended and consequently all the effort put into border molding will come to nothing. Overloading the tray with impression material should be avoided, or it will also cause a thick border.

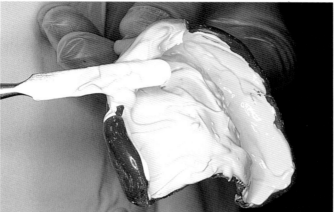

Fig. 9-121 A layer of paste should be smeared on the outer side of the compound border as well as the inside. In this manner the paste will flow out smoothly toward the outside of the tray when the impression is made, and consequently the border will be appropriately recorded.

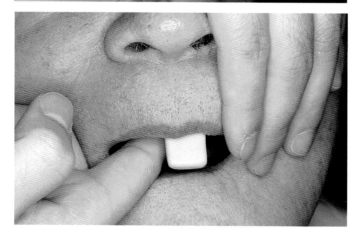

Fig. 9-122 The tray should be seated properly in the mouth and held gently in place. As the details of the mucosa are recorded with the final impression material, when seating the tray in place, care must be taken not to use excessive pressure, otherwise this will result in the fitting surface of the tray coming in direct contact with the mucosa. The lips and cheeks should be gently massaged so that excess material can flow out.

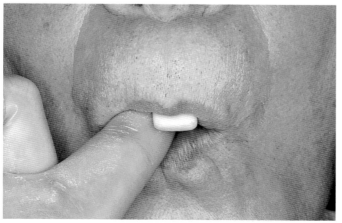

Fig. 9-123 When the material begins to thicken, the patient should be asked to purse the lips and simultaneously, the lips and cheeks should be massaged. The movements of the tissue in function will be recorded in the frenal areas and the round borders covered with a thin layer of paste will also be recorded in all areas.

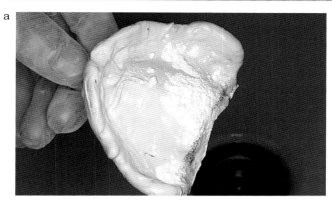

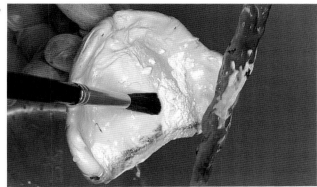

Fig. 1a, b When the impression is removed, a layer of mucous saliva covering the palate often adheres to its surface. The saliva can be easily eliminated by sprinkling plaster over the saliva and then washing it off with tap water. When the thick mucous saliva has displaced the impression material and details of the mucosa are not evident, the saliva on the palate should be wiped off and the impression should be repeated.

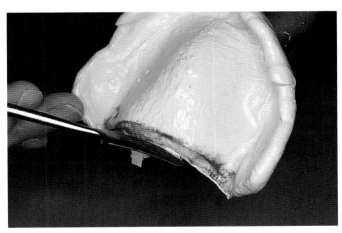

Fig. 9-124 Excess paste that has flowed beyond the posterior border of the tray should be trimmed with a hot spatula.

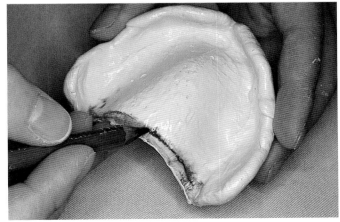

Fig. 9-125 The pencil mark of the ah-line that has been transferred to the impression should be accentuated with an indelible pencil. Consequently, this line can be clearly transferred onto the master cast.

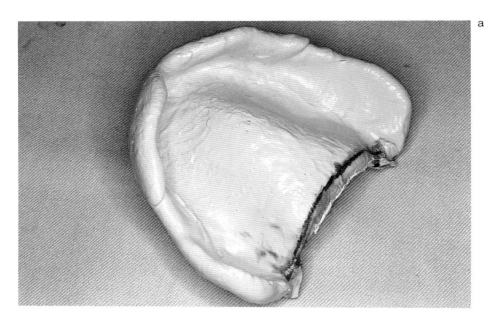

a

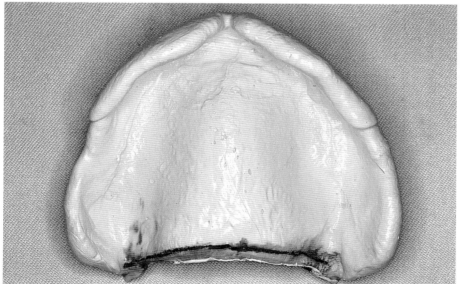

b

Fig. 9-126a, b   The completed final maxillary impression. It is desirable that the tray is evenly covered with a thin layer of impression paste and no local penetration of the tray through the paste appears. However, unless the tray has large exposed areas indicating pressure areas, the impression will be acceptable.

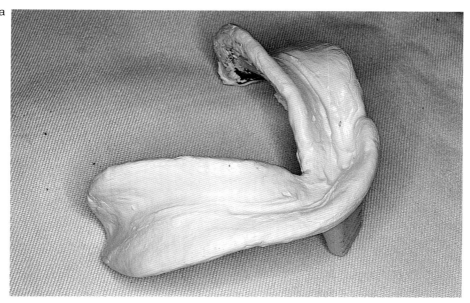

a

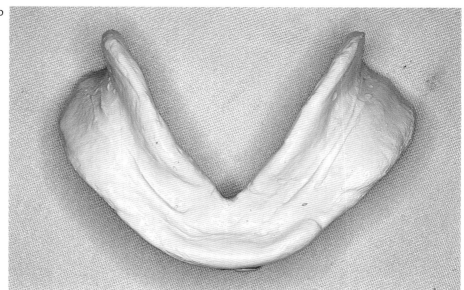

b

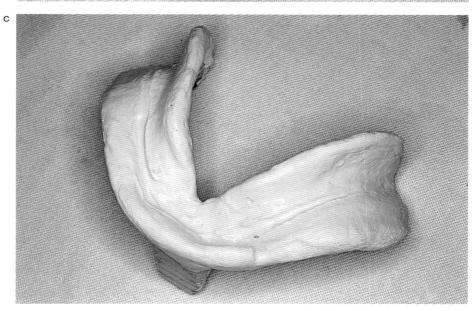

c

Fig. 9-127a~c   The completed final mandibular impression. When the paste begins to thicken, the patient should be instructed to move the tongue to the left and right, and forward to record the lingual frenum in function. These instructions can also prevent the free-flowing impression material from flowing into the floor of the mouth. Nevertheless, when the completed impression is examined, thin overextensions are often found below the borders. These should be trimmed with a sharp knife.

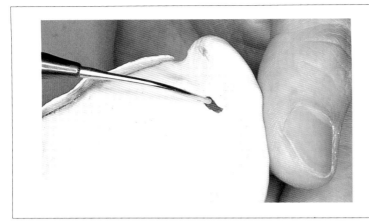

Fig. 1 When an air bubble is found on the impression surface, it should be corrected by the addition of wax. Large air bubbles can be corrected by placing the minimal necessary amount of paste in the deficiency and reseating the impression. Small voids should be disregarded and trimmed off the master cast.

a

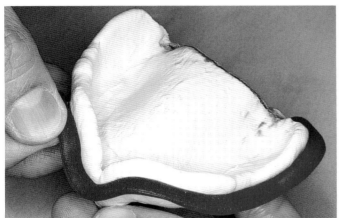

b

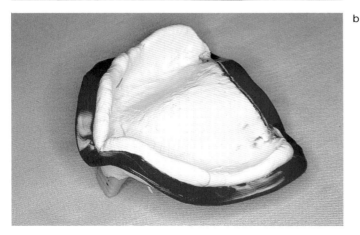

Fig. 9-128a, b Boxing should be performed prior to pouring the cast, to reproduce the impression border precisely on the cast. Even in cases where time is limited, at least beading with utility wax should be done. Beading wax is placed and sealed approximately 3 mm below the border of the impression. Then the beading wax should be flattened by pinching with the fingers to make the land of the cast the proper width. The beading wax should be placed below the surface of the impression across its posterior border, so that the land area of the cast will be above the impression surface of the cast.

a

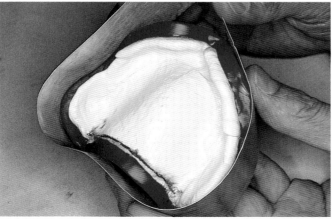

Fig. 9-129a, b A sheet of baseplate wax or lead strip should be folded around the beaded impression to form the base of the cast. It is essential that the boxing strip extends at least 10 mm above the highest point on the impression to provide about 10 mm of stone in the thinnest part for the base. The beading wax should be sealed to the lead strip with a hot spatula to make the seal water tight and strengthen the junction.

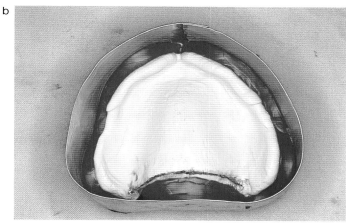

b

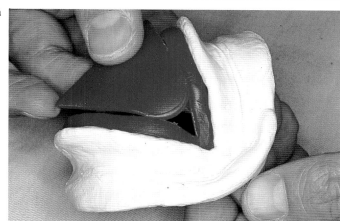

a

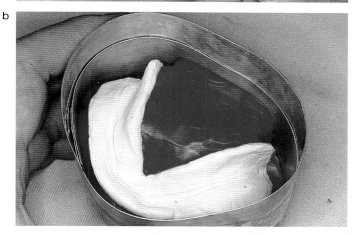

b

Fig. 9-130a, b   After the mandibular impression has been beaded using a similar method to that used for the maxillary impression, the tongue space of the impression should be blocked out by adapting and sealing a sheet of baseplate wax. Extra beading wax should be adapted to the posterior buccal region of the mandibular impression to prevent the land of the cast from being too narrow. Beading wax in the heel area of the mandibular impression should be below the impression.

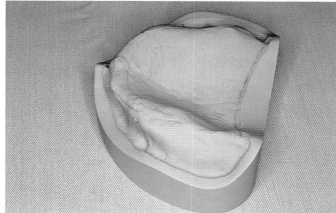

Fig. 9-131   The indelible pencil mark of the ah-line is evident after the cast is separated. The land of the master cast should be 2-3 mm distal to the ah-line in this area. The height of the land in the buccal and labial vestibular areas should be somewhat higher than the widest region (in cross section) of the sulcus.

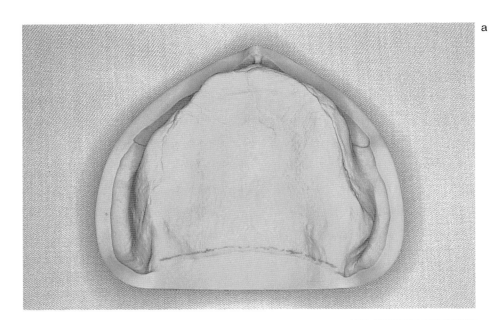

a

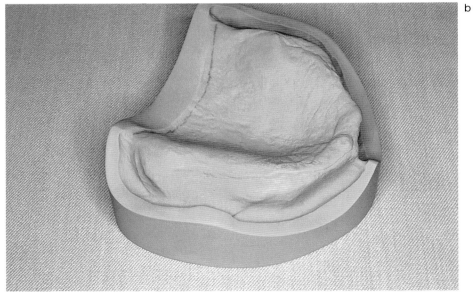

b

Fig. 9-132a, b The completed maxillary master cast. The cast has been adjusted on a model trimmer to make the crest of the ridge nearly parallel to the base. There should be about 10 mm of stone in the thinnest part. Also the sides of the cast should be trimmed so that they are perpendicular to the base.

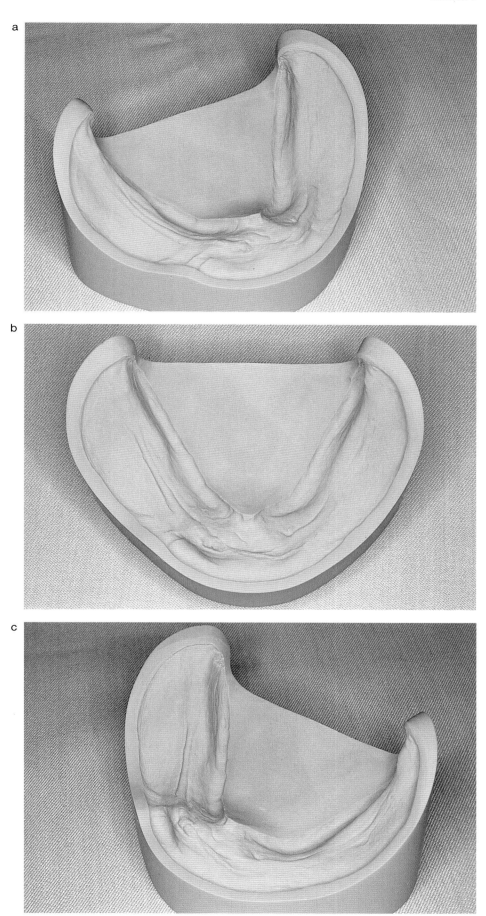

Fig. 9-133a ~ c The completed mandibular master cast.

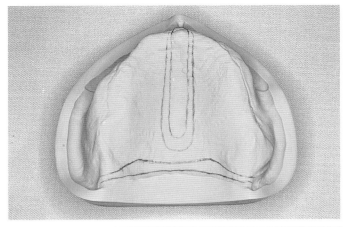

Fig. 9-134 The outlines of the posterior palatal seal(post-dam) and relief areas should be marked with a lead pencil.

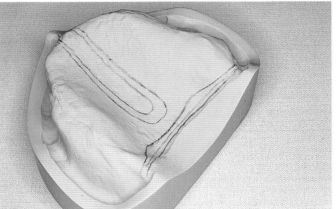

Fig. 9-135 A groove is carved into the cast along the area corresponding with the posterior border region of the denture. The groove should be extended laterally a little beyond the hamular notch. The post-dam is necessary to compensate for the dimensional changes of the denture base resin during polymerization.

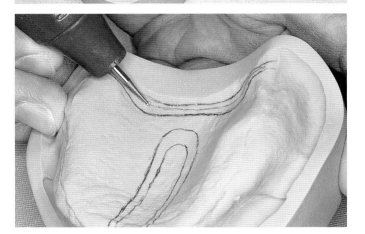

Fig. 9-136 The post-dam is deepest at a point 1/3 of the distance from the posterior edge of the groove and at the midpoint between the midline and hamular notches. It becomes gradually shallower anteroposteriorly and laterally. Using a round bur that is 1.5 mm in diameter, two holes should be drilled to the depth of the bur in the deepest area so as not to carve the post-dam too deeply. They will be used as depth guides for carving the post-dam.

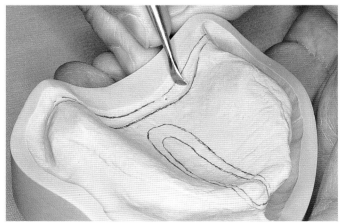

Fig. 9-137 The groove should be carved with a large-sized round bur or a sharp scraper so that it will become gradually shallower anteroposteriorly and laterally from the deepest holes.

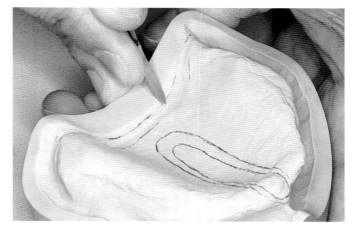

Fig. 9-138   The surfaces of the groove which have been cut should be smoothed with a sharp knife.

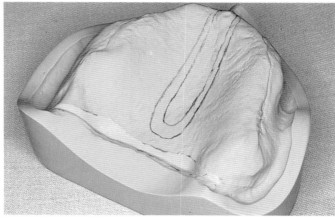

Fig. 9-139   The entire post-dam area has been excavated. In cross-section, it is V-shaped.

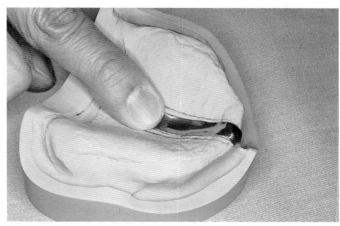

Fig. 9-140   Spiny ridges, torus palatinus, torus mandibularis, etc. are covered with thin mucosa. Metal foil should be placed accordingly on these areas to produce relief on the denture. The area and amount of relief are defined by observation and palpation.

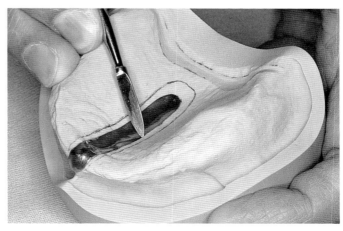

Fig. 9-141   When metal foil is used in two layers, the sides of the inner foil should be tapered and the other layer should be placed on top of the inner one.

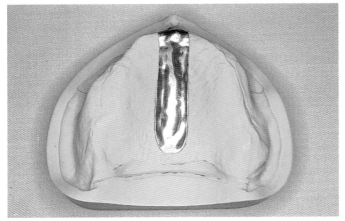

Fig. 9-142 Only after the thickness and resiliency of the mucosa have been incorporated into a cast such as here, does the cast become a "dynamic cast" which represents the actual structures. In areas where the condition of the mucosa can not be clearly detected by palpation, it is better to provide relief using pressure indicating paste at the time of denture insertion.

a

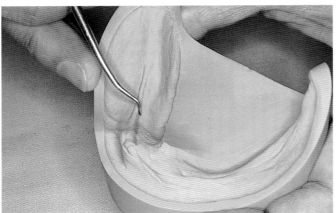

b

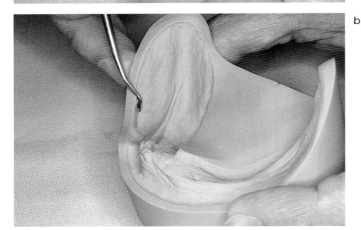

Fig. 9-143a, b Wax should be added into the undercuts and onto the breakable portions prior to baseplate construction. As the mandibular baseplate will be made with an autopolymerizing resin, the cast is liable to break during construction, so this treatment using wax should be carefully done to ensure that the baseplate can be easily removed. However, the amount of wax used should be minimal so as not to spoil the fit of the baseplate.

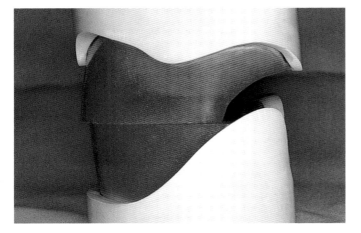

Fig. 9-144 If average dimensions are given to the occlusion rims in advance, the correction during recording jaw relations will be minimized and thus the chairtime will be shortened(cf. p. 50). The upper rim should be somewhat higher and the lower rim lower than their average heights respectively. Usually the dentist finds it easier to remove wax from an upper rim and add wax to a lower rim during the determination of the occlusal plane and the vertical dimension.

Fig. 9-145 Maxillary baseplate and occlusion rim. The maxillary baseplate should be made of shellac baseplate material. Some dentists prefer autopolymerizing resins on the grounds that they are not easily deformed during the recording of the jaw relations. However, the resin in the palatal region must be converted to baseplate wax prior to waxing, leading to a complicated procedure. Also, sometimes the baseplate resin must be cut away to enable the teeth to be set in their proper places. As the final decision regarding the jaw relations is left to the use of a gothic arch tracer, a small deformation of the shellac baseplate does not matter.

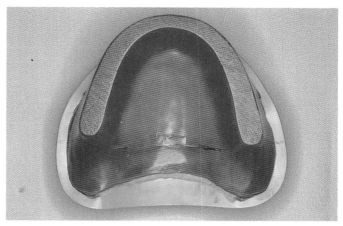

Fig. 9-146 The wax rim should be placed in the position previously occupied by the natural teeth by referring to the landmarks on the cast. Special care should be taken to provide the proper degree of the labial fullness to the maxillary rim. When the labial support is inadequate and thus the appearance is spoiled, it will mislead the determination of the vertical dimension. The labial surface of the rim should be 6-7 mm anterior to the center of the incisive papilla.

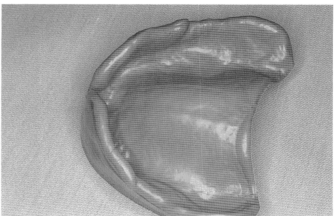

Fig. 9-147 Mandibular baseplate and occlusion rim. This baseplate is made of autopolymerizing resin. In cases with a complicated and irregular ridge form, it is difficult to accurately adapt shellac to the cast. The wax rim should be placed in the position where the natural teeth were situated; in the molar region, in the center of the posterior denture-bearing area buccolingually, and in the anterior region, labially to the so-called alveolar crest. The amount of protrusion should be guessed from the degree of alveolar bone resorption.

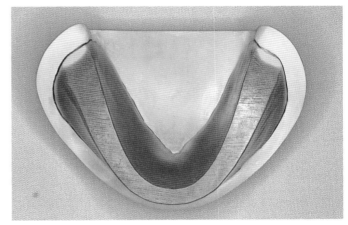

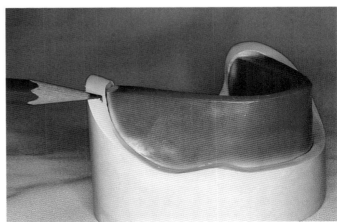

Fig. 9-148 In the molar region of the mandible, the height of the wax rim should be even with the height of the middle of the retromolar pad.

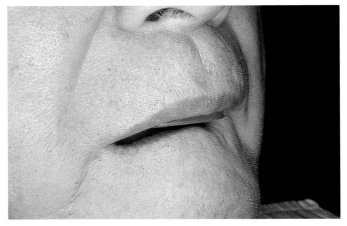

Fig. 9-149 The lower border of the upper wax rim should be even with the lower margin of the upper lip when the patient slightly opens his/her mouth. However, as the length of the upper lip varies with individuals, the lower border of the upper wax rim should be modified after the balance in height between the upper and lower rims has been checked at a later step. At the try-in for the anterior teeth, this level will be finally corrected. If the upper wax rim is not high enough, it must be buit up with extra wax. As adding wax requires much more time than removing wax, the upper wax rim should always be made somewhat higher than its average height.

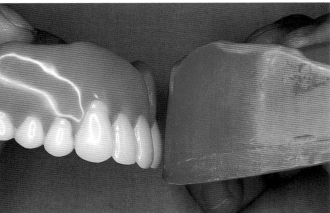

Fig. 9-150 If a patient has existing dentures, they should be inserted into the mouth and the level of the incisal edges of the upper anterior teeth and the labial fullness should be examined. Ideas for improvement can be obtained by referring to the small flaws in the existing denture.

a

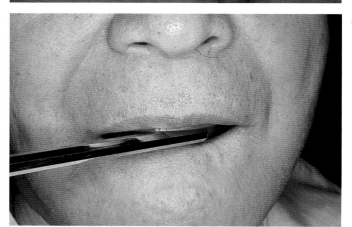

b

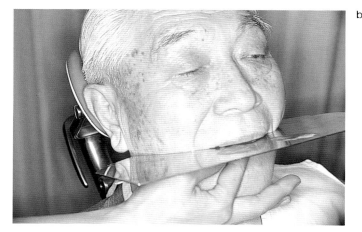

Fig. 9-151a, b After the level of the upper rim in the anterior region has been decided, the position of the occlusal plane in relation to the face should be assessed using an occlusal plane guide. The wax rim should be trimmed so that the occlusal plane is parallel to the interpupillary line when viewed from the front and also parallel to the ala-tragus line when viewed from the side.

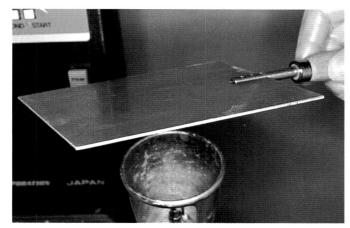

Fig. 9-152 At first, the wax rim should be trimmed with a knife so that the occlusal plane is roughly parallel to the reference plane. A flat metal plate for establishing the occlusal plane is useful to efficiently level the cut surface.

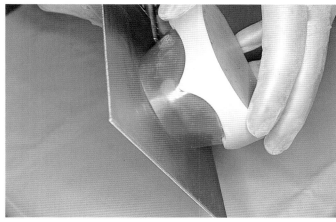

Fig. 9-153 The heated plate should be lightly pressed onto the roughened surface to level it.

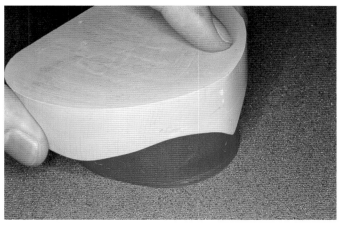

Fig. 9-154 The occlusal plane should then be smoothed by rubbing it on rough sandpaper placed on a flat plane. While this is being done, the rim must be placed on the cast to avoid deformation of the baseplate and the occlusion rim.

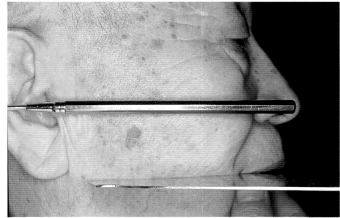

Fig. 9-155 The upper rim has been trimmed so that the occlusal plane is approximately parallel with the ala-tragus line. After that, the occlusal plane should be adjusted slightly by referring to the amount of alveolar bone resorption and the space that is needed for setting the teeth.

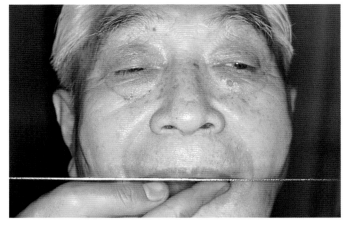

Fig. 9-156 The occlusal plane is parallel to the interpupillary line when viewed from the front. The earlobes, as well as the interpupillary line, are a useful guide when leveling the occlusal plane. The balance of the heights of the right and left sides of the occlusion rim obtained in this way will not need further major adjustment.

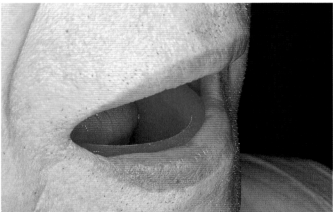
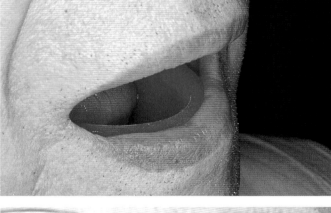

Fig. 9-157 The upper border of the mandibular wax rim should be even with the upper margin of the lower lip when the patient slightly opens his/her mouth.

a

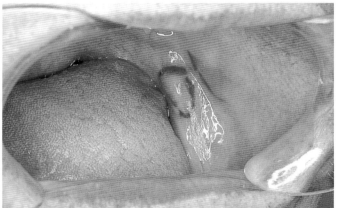

b

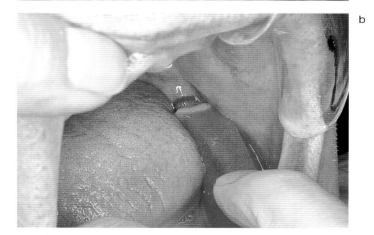

Fig. 9-158a, b The retromolar pad should be circled. The mandibular occlusion rim should be inserted into the mouth and its height in the molar region should be assessed by referring to the pad. The height of the rim should be even with the level of the middle of the pad. As the temporalis muscle fibers attach to the distal portion of the retromolar pad, stimulation from this muscle prevents the pad from resorbing. Therefore the pad is useful for orientating the occlusal plane. Also, the level of the dorsum of the tongue can be used as a guide for orientation of the occlusal plane.

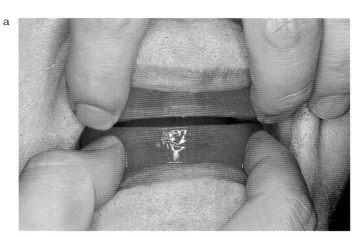

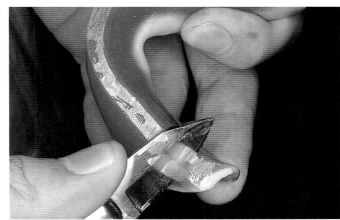

Fig. 9-159a, b Both rims should be inserted into the mouth and held firmly in place with the fingers. The patient should then be instructed to close the rims together and the degree of contact should be observed with the lips retracted by the fingers. In this case, there is a premature contact in the left posterior region. The lower wax rim should be trimmed so that it meets the upper rim approximately evenly. However, sometimes readjustment of the upper rim may be required to correct an imbalance in height between the upper and lower rims.

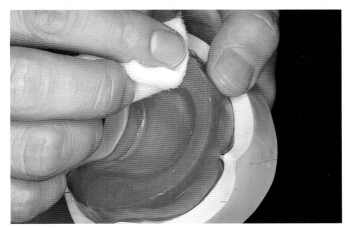

Fig. 9-160 The upper occlusion rim should be coated with a separating medium such as vaseline to avoid adhesion to the softened lower rim at the next step.

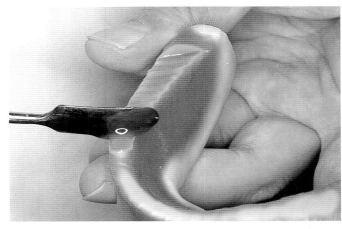

Fig. 9-161 The surface of the lower occlusion rim should be evenly softened by tapping all over it with the edge of a heated wax spatula.

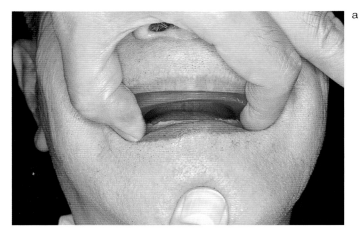

a

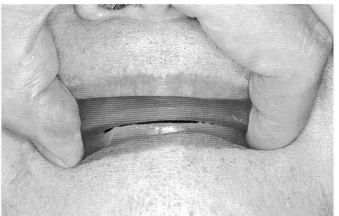

b

Fig. 9-162a, b Instruct the patient to close gently, lightly guiding the mandible posteriorly with the right thumb and index finger holding the chin. At the same time, the thumb and index finger of the other hand are used to hold the lower occlusion rim in place, which then slides gently on the soft surface of the fingers as the mouth is closed. This method enables the dentist to check visually and by tactile sensation whether or not the contact between the upper and lower rims is even.

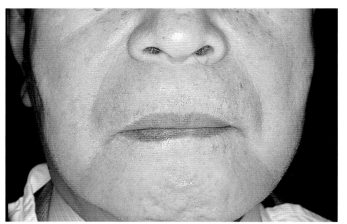

Fig. 9-163 When even contact is obtained, the patient's appearance should be carefully observed. If the occlusal vertical dimension is too great, the lower third of the face will appear longer and the lips will be incompetent. If too small, the vermilion border will become thin and wrinkles will occur on the lips. The chin will have a protruded appearance. The occlusal vertical dimension is adequate when recorded between the above two situations.

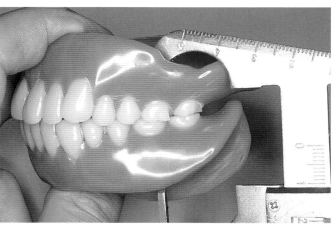

Fig. 9-164 If there are existing dentures, by using the information obtained from them, the occlusal vertical dimension can be determined quickly and easily. The upper and lower dentures should be put into occlusion with each other outside the mouth and the distance between the fitting surfaces corresponding with the crests of the upper and lower ridges at some point in the posterior region should be measured with calipers. The occlusal vertical dimension of the new dentures must be greater than this value. By referring to the amount of tooth abrasion of the old dentures and amount of bone resorption, we can estimate by how much we should increase the occlusal vertical dimension. Of course, the patient's appearance with dentures can also help this estimation.

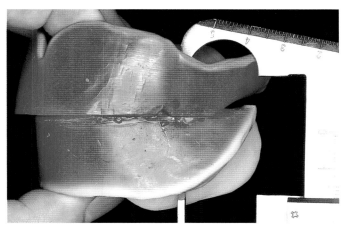

Fig. 9-165 The rims, which meet evenly, should be removed from the mouth and the distance between the fitting surfaces of the upper and lower rims should be measured at the same point as was measured on the existing dentures. In this case, the value is a little greater than the estimated occlusal vertical dimension. Repeat the above procedure until the estimated height has been achieved.

a

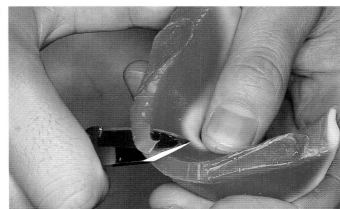

b

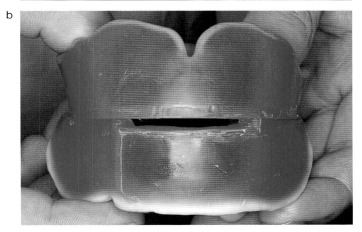

Fig. 9-166a,b Remove wax from the surface of the lower rim in the anterior region as much as is required to reduce the vertical occlusal dimension. The cutout space in the anterior region serves as a guide for the dentist to stop the closure when the patient closes onto the softened lower rim. The lower rim should not come into contact with the upper rim anteriorly when recording the jaw relations. If contact between the rims occurs, there may be displacement of the rims or a shift of the mandible out of the centric occlusal position.

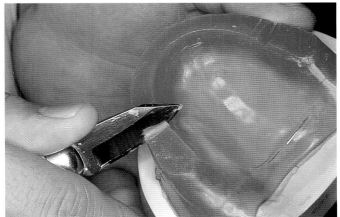

Fig. 9-167 V-shaped notches should be cut on both sides of the upper rim to locate the rims exactly.

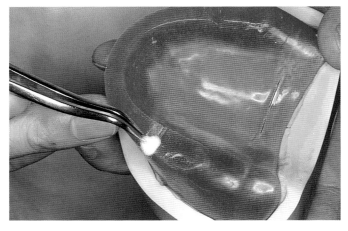

Fig. 9-168   The V-shaped notches should be smeared with a very thin layer of vaseline.

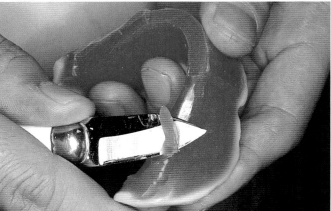

Fig. 9-169   Before softening the occlusal plane of the lower occlusion rim, it should be trimmed buccally and lingually to form a peak in cross-section.

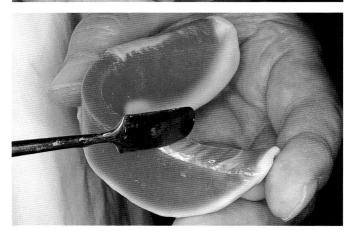

Fig. 9-170   When the surface of the rim is softened by tapping it with the edge of a heated wax spatula, the peak-shaped rim facilitates the transfer of heat and enables the dentist to evenly soften the wax for a short time.

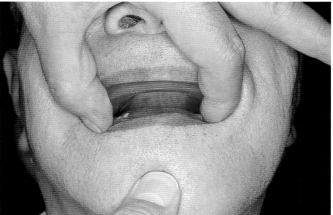

Fig. 9-171   As the final decision of the horizontal jaw relation is left to the use of the gothic arch tracer, at this step the recording of the vertical jaw relation will be established and the horizontal jaw relation will be roughly recorded. It requires great skill to simultaneously record the horizontal and vertical jaw relations using the rims to establish an exact jaw relationship. If one appointment is used just for recording the vertical jaw relation, the recording can be easily performed and chairtime will be reduced.

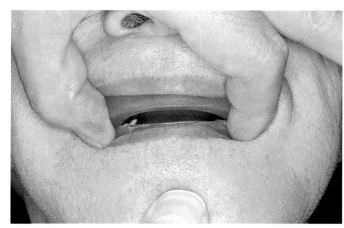

Fig. 9-172   Instruct the patient to close gently, lightly guiding the mandible posteriorly using the same technique as that used in Fig. 9-162. This is done by saying to the patient, "Close on your back teeth". If the thumb is not placed against the chin, most patients will close anteriorly to the centric occlusal position. However, strong pressure should not be used on the chin, otherwise the jaw will protrude. Also, pushing back the corners of the mouth with the fingers helps guide the mandible posteriorly during closure.

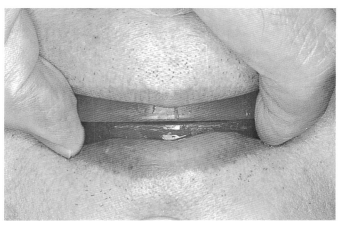

Fig. 9-173   If contact between the rims occurs in the anterior region whilst recording the jaw relation, it may cause displacement of the rims or shift of the mandible out of the centric occlusal position. So, closure should be stopped when the lower rim is just short of contact with the upper rim.

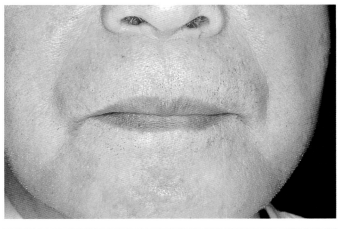

Fig. 9-174   Regarding the amount of protrusion of the upper rim, as an average degree has been provided by referring to the incisive papilla, there is no need to significantly correct it. The labial fullness of the upper lip should be finally checked when the occlusal vertical dimension has been decided. In this case the upper lip looks slightly too prominent.

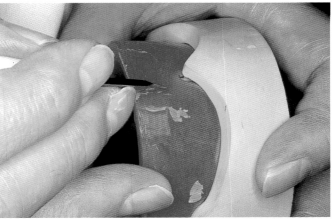

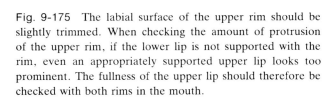

Fig. 9-175   The labial surface of the upper rim should be slightly trimmed. When checking the amount of protrusion of the upper rim, if the lower lip is not supported with the rim, even an appropriately supported upper lip looks too prominent. The fullness of the upper lip should therefore be checked with both rims in the mouth.

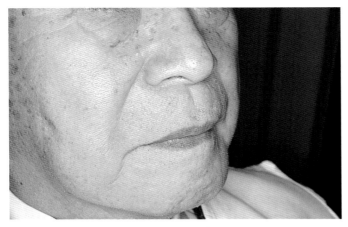

Fig. 9-176 The patient's appearance after completing the jaw registration. Facial contours, as well as the fullness of the lips and cheeks, should be examined from in front of the face and in profile.

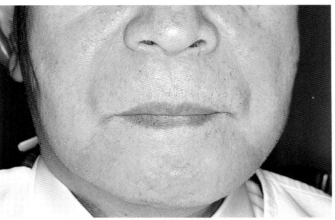

Fig. 9-177 The lips are properly supported, no wrinkles appear on the upper lip and the nasolabial folds have an appropriate depth, leading to a natural appearance. Also, the chin is not apparently protruded.

a

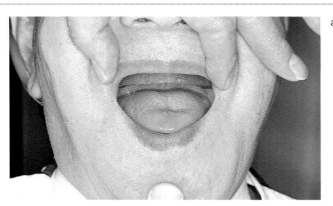

b

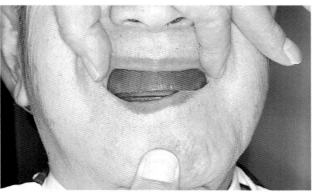

Fig. 1a, b If patients are strained, they tend to protrude the mandible or sometimes cannot even move it at all. This situation makes it difficult for the dentist to guide the mandible. However, when the operator's guidance with the fingers is repeated, the patient and even the dentist will become tired, and at that time the tension will be relieved. Then, the dentist will be able to record the centric occlusal position. However, it is time-consuming. In this case, the patient should be instructed to open wide and then close while the dentist pushes the chin posteriorly. When the condyles drop into the glenoid fossae with a slight "clicking" sensation, if the patient is allowed to finish closing the mouth, the patient will close his/her mandible into the centric occlusal position.

Fig. 1 The author determines the occlusal vertical dimension by referring to the morphological harmony of the face, namely the appearance(p.52). However, physiological methods, especially the method using the rest position of the mandible, seem to be commonly used for determining the occlusal vertical dimension. Functional methods are effective, but they are affected by the skill, mental tension and posture of the patient, which can easily lead to errors. No method can give a perfect indication for determining the occlusal vertical dimension. The dentist may be helped due to the wide permissible range for the vertical relation.

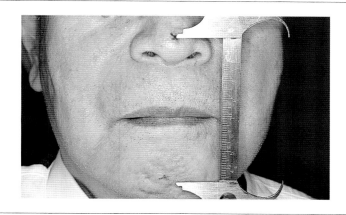

Fig. 9-178 The midline of the mouth should be scored with a knife on the occlusion rim. The knife should be placed below the labial frenum and then the midline should be marked by considering the overall balance of the face by referring to the philtrum of the lip and the midline of the face. This position may be slightly adjusted during the try-in procedure for the anterior teeth.

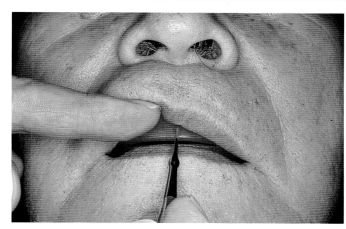

Fig. 9-179 Marks should be scored on the rim at the corners of the mouth, or vertical lines should be extended from the lateral surfaces of the alae of the nose onto the labial surface of the rim. The former indicates the location of the distal surface of the upper canine and the latter indicates the position of its apex. The distance between the alae marks or the distance between the marks made at the corners of the mouth will provide an indication of the width of the upper anterior teeth. However, these are not entirely reliable for using as a guide for the selection of the upper anterior teeth.

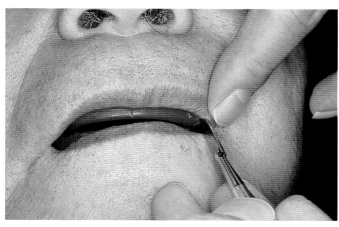

a

Fig. 9-180a, b The high and low lip lines should be scored on the labial surfaces of the rims. The high lip line indicates the highest position of the upper lip and the low lip line indicates the lowest position of the lower lip when the patient is instructed to say "ee..." strongly. These serve as a guide for determining the length of the anterior teeth. Also it is essential to arrange the upper and lower anterior teeth in a well balanced fashion between these two lines.

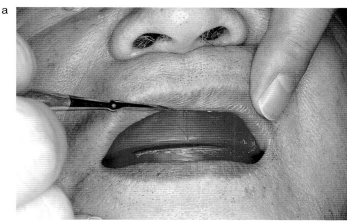

b

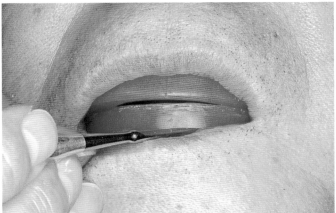

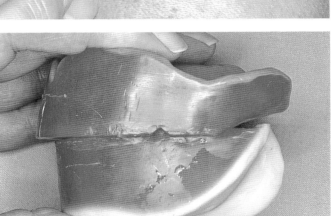

Fig. 9-181 The upper and lower rims removed from the mouth should be related according to the interocclusal record and their relationship should be checked. Sometimes the posterior border of the lower baseplate may collide with the upper rim. In such a case, as the wax rims may have been displaced during recording, the premature contact should be removed by trimming the wax rim or the baseplate and the jaw registration should be performed again.

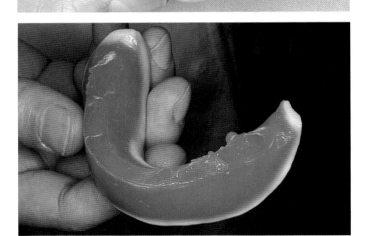

Fig. 9-182 Sometimes an extra material such as zinc oxide-eugenol paste is used as the recording medium to make the jaw registration more precise. However, this is not necessary because the final decision with regard to the horizontal jaw relation will be performed using the gothic arch tracer. This step is preliminary, and so a wax record can be made without using any extra material.

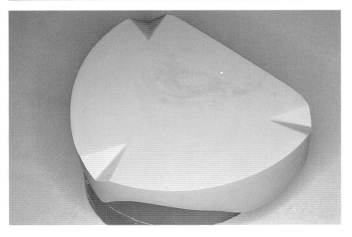

Fig. 9-183 In order to accurately replace the cast on the articulator after processing, prior to mounting the cast, for indexing, V-shaped notches should be carved in the base of the cast. The surface of the base should be smoothed with sandpaper and then the notches should be placed in thicker portions of the cast so as to avoid breakage.

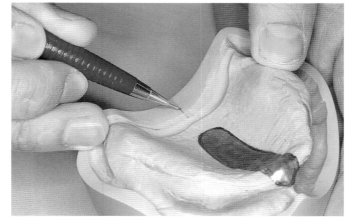

Fig. 9-184 The midline of the upper cast should be marked on the posterior land of the cast by referring to the foveae palatinae etc.

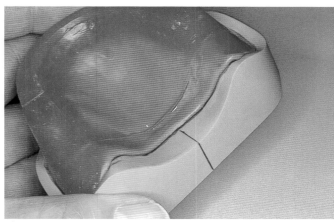

Fig. 9-185 This line should be extended onto the side and base of the cast.

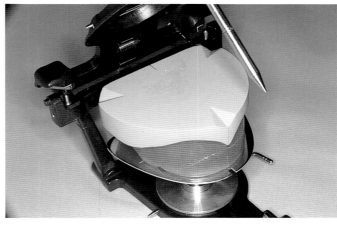

Fig. 9-186 Place the maxillary cast and occlusion rim on the occlusal plane table placed on the lower frame of the articulator. The cast should be positioned so that the midline of the occlusion rim is aligned with the tip of the incisal indicator pin anteriorly and the line drawn on the base(Fig. 9-185) is aligned with the mark indicating the midline in front of the spring of the articulator posteriorly. The articulator should be closed and the clearance between the cast and the upper frame should be checked.

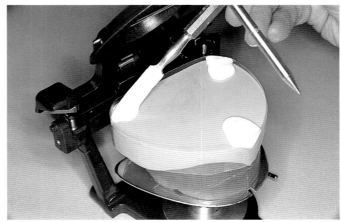

Fig. 9-187 The basal surface of the cast should be painted with a separating medium and a strip of vinyl tape should be wrapped around the cast to confine the stone. The cast and occlusion rim should be replaced on the occlusal plane table and the wax rim should then be temporarily fixed to the table with wax. Stone should be placed on the top of the cast. The notches should be carefully filled with stone.

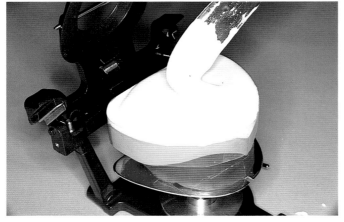

Fig. 9-188 As the height of the vinyl tape has been trimmed according to the clearance between the cast and the upper frame of the articulator, the boxed space should be filled with artificial stone. The cast can be mounted with plaster, but stone is preferable because of its reduced setting expansion.

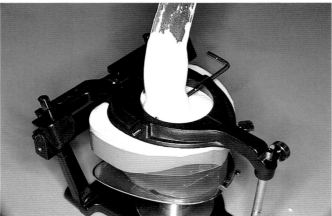

Fig. 9-189 The articulator should be closed and additional stone should be placed through the hole in the upper frame. The frame should be gently tapped with the handle of a plaster spatula to distribute the stone evenly under the frame.

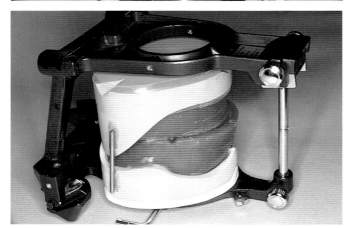

Fig. 9-190 After the stone has set, the articulator should be placed upside down to mount the lower cast. The lower cast should be related to the upper cast using an interocclusal record and then they should be firmly joined together with steel rods and sticky wax.

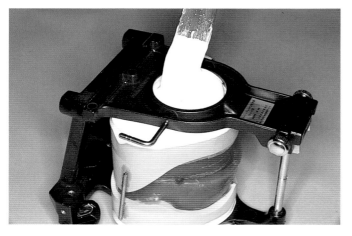

Fig. 9-191 The lower cast should be boxed with a strip of vinyl tape and stone should be placed on its base using a similar technique to that used for the upper cast. As the lower cast will be finally mounted after the horizontal jaw relation is recorded using the gothic arch tracer, at this step the cast can be temporarily attached to the articulator with impression plaster which has a fast setting time.

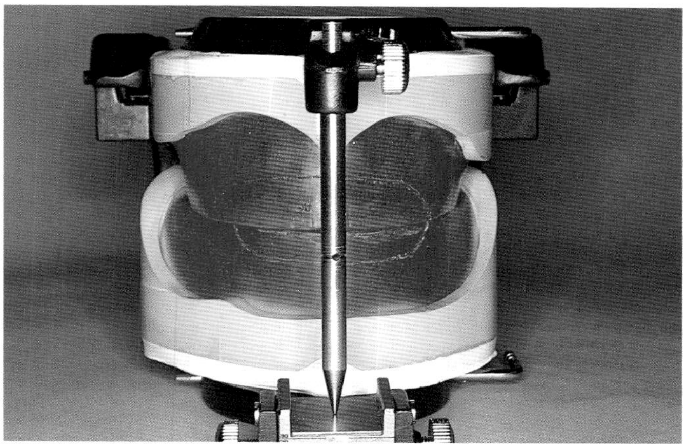

Fig. 9-192 After the stone has set, make certain that the incisal pin comes in contact with the incisal guide table. The vinyl tape should be removed and the mounting stone trimmed. Regarding the upper cast, make certain that it can be separated from the mounting stone and then it should be replaced on the articulator by means of the notches. The cast should be joined to the mounting stone again by sticking vinyl tape along the junction.

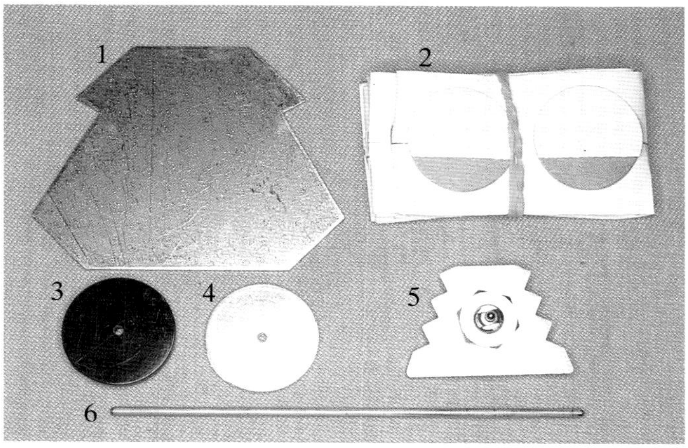

Fig. 9-193 Gothic arch tracer (The simplex intra-oral gothic arch tracer, Dentsply). 1. tracing plate , 2. adhesive tape, 3. stylus positioning disc, 4. centric lock disc, 5. stylus assembly, 6. disc positioning needle.

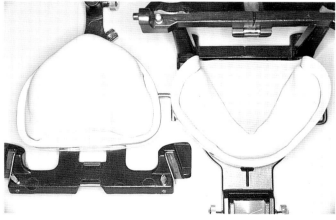

Fig. 9-194 The baseplates and occlusion rims should be removed from the casts on the articulator and then the record bases should be constructed on the casts. The record bases should be made of autopolymerizing resin to minimize their deformation when recording the jaw relations. The record base should be well adapted to the cast and given the same border contour as the denture will have. This will ensure the base will not be displaced during jaw registration. Its thickness should be approximately even all over the cast. The desired thickness is approximately 2 mm.

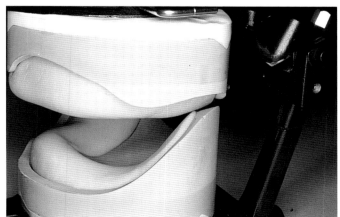

Fig. 9-195 Close the articulator and make certain that there is no contact between the upper and lower record bases, especially in the posterior region. In this case, they contact each other in the posterior region, so the contact should be eliminated by trimming each base.

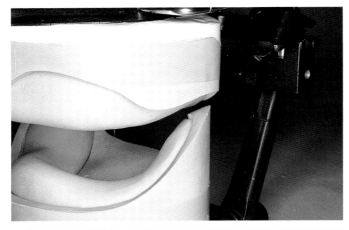

Fig. 9-196 As the relationship between the upper and lower bases will be somewhat different in the mouth and also the mandible will move during jaw registration, a rather wide clearance should be provided between the upper and lower record bases.

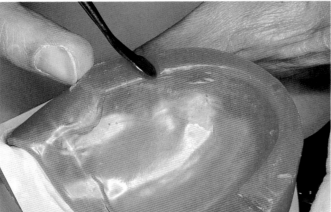

Fig. 9-197 The upper occlusion rim should be replaced onto the cast and the V-shaped notches previously carved in the rim should be filled with melted wax and made level with the occlusal plane.

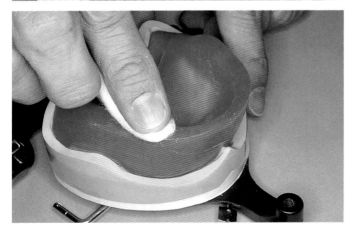

Fig. 9-198 The occlusal plane should be coated with a separating medium, such as vaseline.

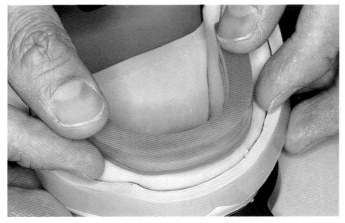

Fig. 9-199a, b A softened horseshoe-shaped wax block should be placed on the lower record base and the articulator should be closed.

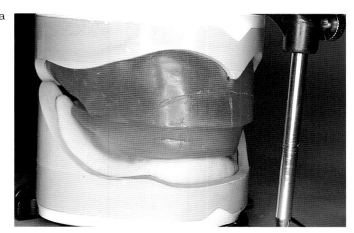

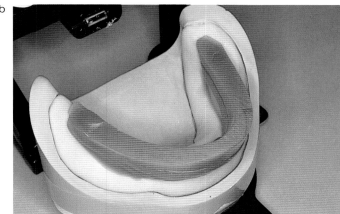

Fig. 9-200a, b The occlusal plane of the upper rim has been transferred onto the lower wax rim. Instead of this record base and rim, the lower baseplate and rim previously used can also be used for the gothic arch tracing method.

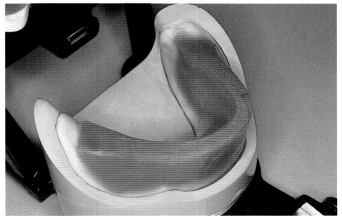

Fig. 9-201 The wax rim should be reinforced by adding extra wax onto its lingual and buccal surfaces. The wax should be sealed to the record base with a hot spatula and smoothed toward the periphery. The occlusal surface of the record rim should be leveled by trimming any excess wax protruding from the transferred occlusal plane.

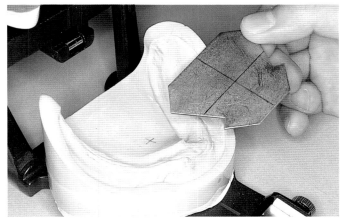

Fig. 9-202 The lower cast and tracing table should be marked anteroposteriorly and laterally to find the center points. These center points will be used for centering the stylus assembly.

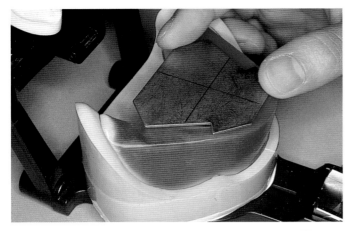

Fig. 9-203 The tracing table should be positioned on the wax rim so that the center point of the tracing table is vertically aligned with the center point of the cast.

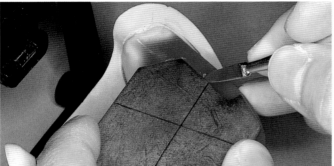

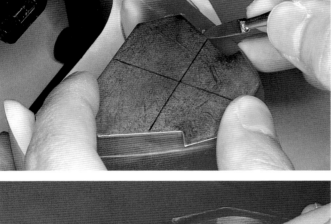

Fig. 9-204 The outline of the tracing plate should be scored with a knife on the occlusal surface of the lower wax rim.

Fig. 9-205 The height of the tracing table should be level with the occlusal plane of the wax rim. The wax inside the outline of the tracing table, approximately half the thickness of the tracing plate, should be removed. This will serve as a guide when positioning the plate in place.

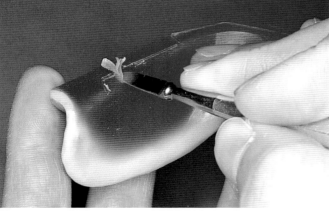

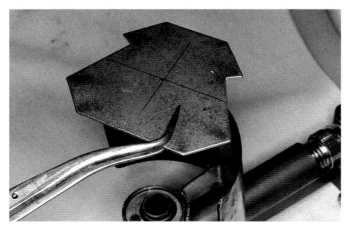

Fig. 9-206 The tracing plate should be warmed over a Bunsen burner. If it is overheated, it will sink too far into the wax when placed on the wax rim.

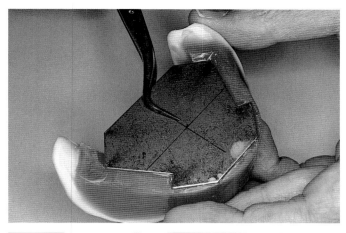

Fig. 9-207 The warmed tracing plate should be gently placed on the cut-out area of the wax rim. Its position should be finely adjusted so that the tracing table is aligned with the occlusal plane. Excess wax around the tracing plate should be removed and then smoothed level with the occlusal plane.

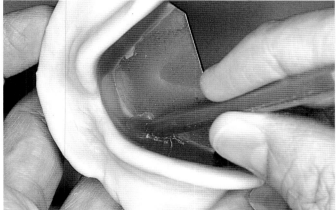

Fig. 9-208 The tracing plate has been fixed to the wax rim with baseplate wax as shown in Fig. 9-207. However, there is the possibility that the tracing plate will be removed by the force of the tongue confined under the plate during the jaw registration. Therefore the tracing plate should be sealed to the wax rim on the underside with sticky wax to make a strong junction.

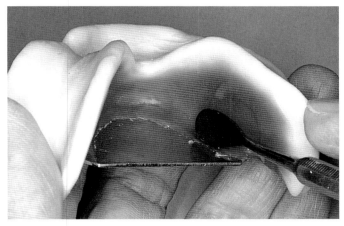

Fig. 9-209 The surface of the sticky wax should be smoothed with a hot spatula to diminish any discomfort for the patient during the jaw registration.

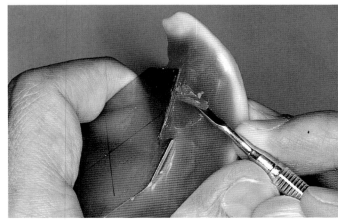

Fig. 9-210 Trim the wax along the outer edges of the tracing plate, bevelling it toward the periphery. It will provide a positive index for a plaster interocclusal record.

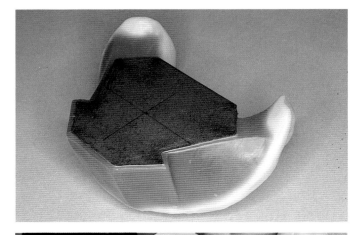

Fig. 9-211 At this time, there should be a little bit of wax remaining(1-1.5 mm in width) beyond the border of the plate. As the wax left around the plate grasps the plate, the strong connection will not be spoiled.

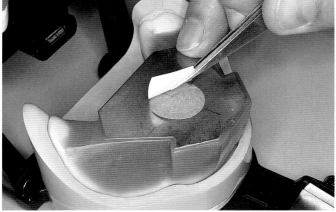

Fig. 9-212 A disc of double-sided adhesive tape should be placed at the approximate center of the tracing table.

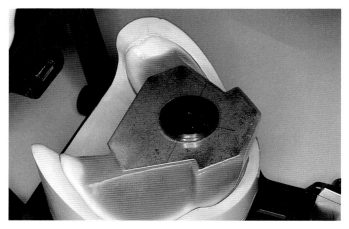

Fig. 9-213 The black disc(stylus positioning disc) should be placed on the adhesive tape so that the hole in the disc is aligned with the center mark of the tracing table.

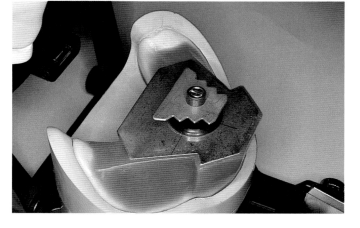

Fig. 9-214 The stylus should be placed in the hole of the disc. The articulator should be closed to make certain that the incisal pin comes into contact with the incisal table. If contact between them is not obtained due to collision between the record base and the stylus assembly, this should be eliminated by trimming the record base. Even though the record base is trimmed, if there is not enough space for the stylus assembly, it must be shifted somewhat posteriorly.

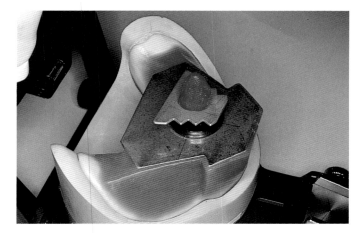

Fig. 9-215 After ascertaining that there are no interferences with the upper record base, a cone of utility wax should be placed on top of the stylus assembly.

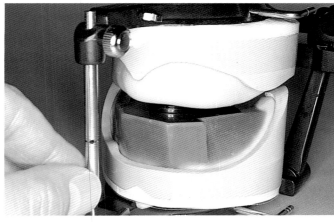

Fig. 9-216 The articulator should be slowly closed until contact is made between the incisal guide pin and the incisal guide table. The occlusal vertical dimension determined with the occlusion rims has been transferred to the Gothic arch tracer assembly and is maintained between the stylus and the tracing table.

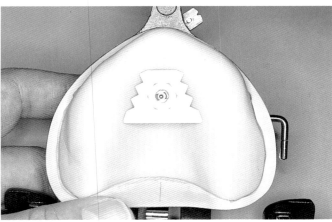

Fig. 9-217 When the articulator is gently opened, the stylus assembly has become attached to the palatal area of the upper record base with the utility wax.

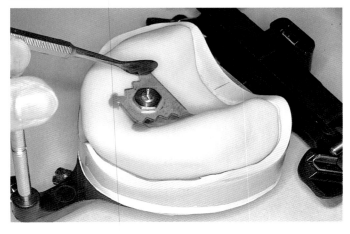

Fig. 9-218 The corners of the stylus assembly should be fixed to the record base with sticky wax, taking care not to displace the stylus assembly.

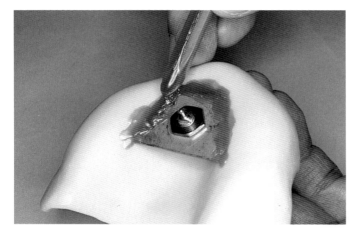

Fig. 9-219 The upper record base should be removed from the cast and the stylus assembly should be firmly fixed by adding sticky wax around the stylus assembly. The surface of the sticky wax should be smoothed with a hot spatula.

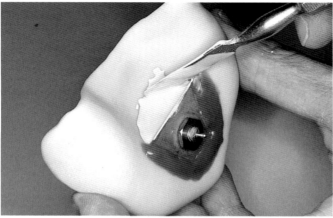

Fig. 9-220 An attachment using only sticky wax will lead to a weak connection, resulting in the stylus assembly being raised and displaced by the pressure that the patient exerts during jaw registration. Thus plaster should be added into the space between the stylus assembly and the record base to strengthen the support of the stylus assembly.

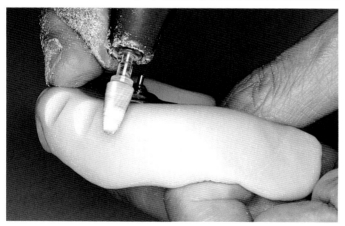

Fig. 9-221 Notches should be ground on the labial surface of the upper record base with a bur. These notches will provide an index for a plaster interocclusal record.

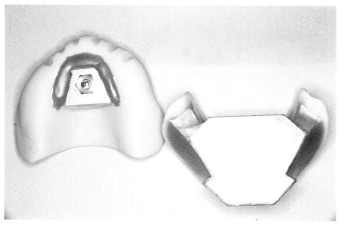

Fig. 9-222 The gothic arch tracer attached to the upper and lower record bases.

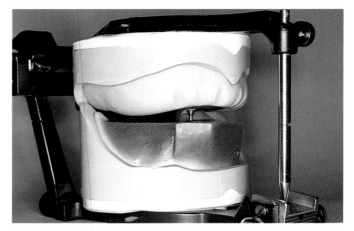

Fig. 9-223 Close the articulator and ensure that the stylus comes into contact with the tracing table. If there is no contact, the stylus screw should be adjusted until contact is made between them.

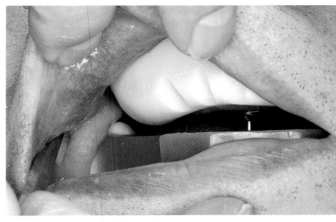

Fig. 9-224 When the patient moves the mandible laterally and anteroposteriorly with the stylus in contact with the tracing table, make certain that the upper and lower record bases do not interfere with each other. If there is any interference, this should be eliminated.

a

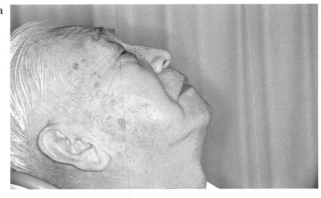

b

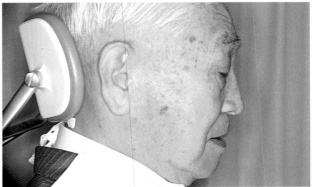

Fig. 1a, b If the patient's head is tilted forward or backward excessively, a correct record cannot be obtained. Jaw registration should be performed with the patient upright and with the head in line with the trunk.

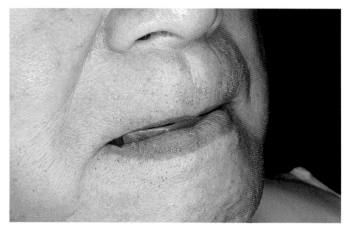

Fig. 9-225 The patient should be instructed to repeatedly move the mandible anteroposteriorly and laterally with the stylus and the tracing table in contact with each other. Some patients cannot understand the dentist's instructions for moving the jaw and cannot move the mandible well. In such a case, the patient should be instructed to move the mandible while looking in a mirror. This facilitates the patient's understanding of the proper jaw movements, leading to the desired movements.

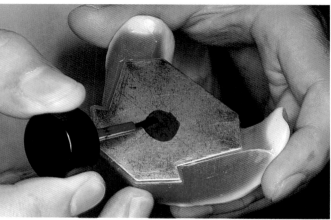

Fig. 9-226 After the patient has mastered moving the mandible smoothly, the needle point tracing faintly drawn on the tracing table with the stylus should be covered with tracing ink.

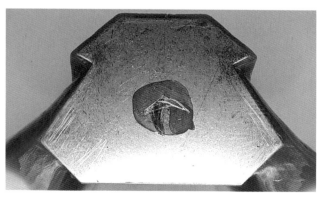

Fig. 1 The mandible should first be protruded, then retruded to the most retruded position and moved laterally. The left and right lateral movements should not be done in succession and should be made separately after the jaw is protruded and retruded. Otherwise, a dull or round apex will occur on the tracing.

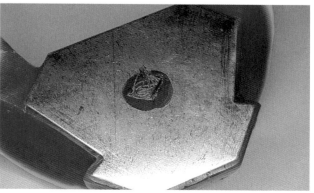

Fig. 2 In spite of repeated instruction and training, some patients cannot make a needle point tracing. In such a case, the patient should be instructed to freely move the mandible. A diamond shape which represents the extreme positions into which the mandible can move will be drawn and the apex indicates the retruded position of the mandible.

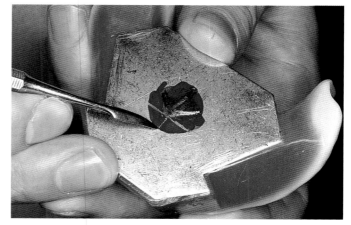

Fig. 9-227 After Gothic arch tracings have been made by the border movements of the mandible, the position of the apex should be registered by drawing additional lines in the ink.

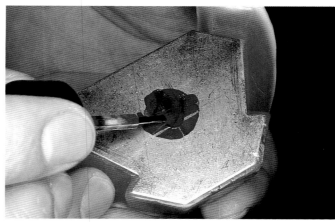

Fig. 9-228 Tracing ink should be painted on the Gothic arch tracings so that they disappear. However, the position of the apex can be guessed by referring to the additional lines.

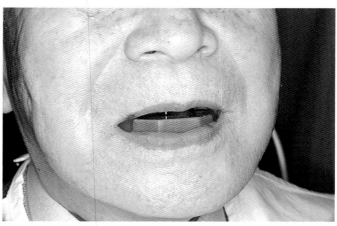

Fig. 9-229 The patient should be instructed to repeat light opening and closing movements in the molar region after reinserting the Gothic arch tracer assembly into the mouth.

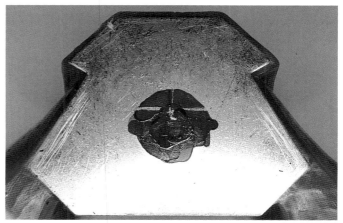

Fig. 9-230 The points made by the light tapping movements are scattered at first, but when the patient becomes accustomed to this procedure and the muscles become relaxed, the scattered points gradually become focused to form a single point. When the scattered points have become focused onto one point, this signals that the centric occlusal position has been recorded.

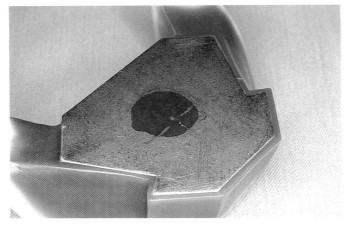

Fig. 9-231 The relative positions of the tapping point and the apex of the Gothic arch tracings should be examined. In this case, the tapping point is located slightly anterior to the apex. So an interocclusal record can be made using this tapping point. In cases with a "habitual eccentric occlusion", the two points may be far apart and so it will be necessary to correct it gradually using treatment dentures.

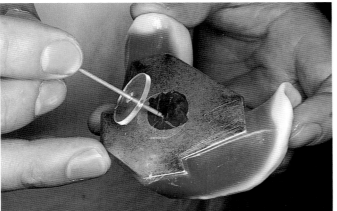

Fig. 9-232 A disc of adhesive tape should be placed on the tracing table so that the center of the disc is aligned with the tapping point. The tapping point is clearly visible through the disc. The centric lock disc with the bevelled portion of the hole facing upward should be placed on the disc positioning needle and then the point of the positioning needle placed exactly onto the tapping point. The disc should be lowered and pressed firmly onto the adhesive tape.

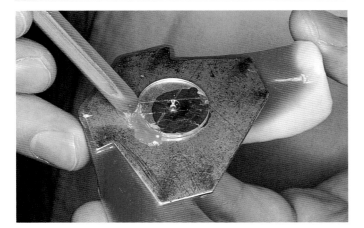

Fig. 9-233 The centric lock disc should be sealed with sticky wax so that it is not displaced whilst making a plaster interocclusal record.

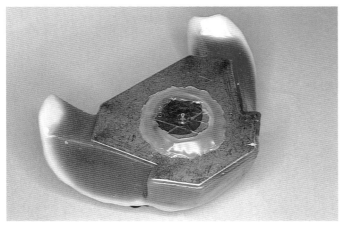

Fig. 9-234 The surface of the sticky wax should be smoothed with a hot spatula so that the plaster interocclusal record can be replaced in its original position when mounting the lower cast using the record.

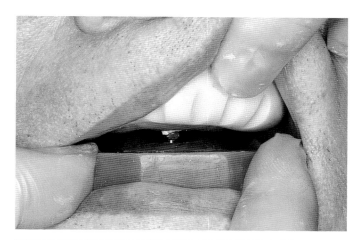

Fig. 9-235　The upper and lower record bases should be reinserted into the mouth. The patient should be instructed to gently close so that the stylus drops into the hole of the centric lock disc. This step requires some mandibular guidance by the dentist. It is important to make certain that the stylus has been exactly placed in the hole.

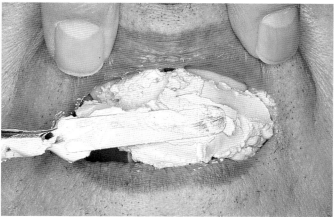

Fig. 9-236　This position should be held with just enough pressure to maintain contact between the stylus and the tracing table. Fast setting plaster should be placed between the upper and lower record bases with a disposable syringe.

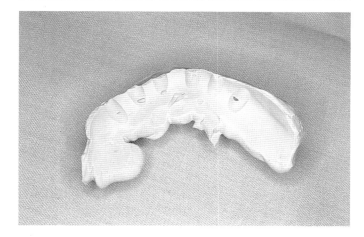

Fig. 9-237　The plaster should be added as required to sufficiently fill the indexing grooves of the upper record base and the indexes around the tracing table.

Fig. 9-238a, b　After the plaster forming the interocclusal record has set, the patient should be instructed to open the mouth carefully, and the tracing assembly and the interocclusal record should be removed as one unit. Then they should be carefully separated. Alternatively, they may be removed separately from the mouth. However, in this case, much more care must be taken so as not to break the plaster interocclusal record.

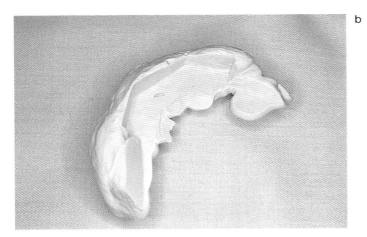

b

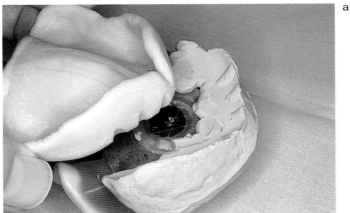

a

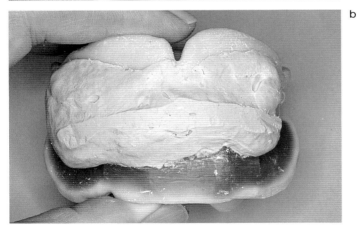

b

Fig. 9-239a, b The upper and lower record bases should be put together again using the plaster interocclusal record. Check that the plaster interocclusal record seats correctly in the indexes of the record bases. The interocclusal record must have enough bulk to join the record bases accurately.

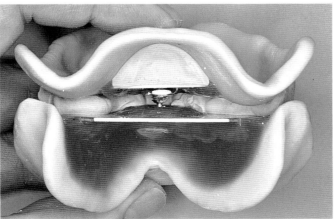

Fig. 9-240 Make certain that the stylus drops into the hole of the centric lock disc by observing the record bases from the rear.

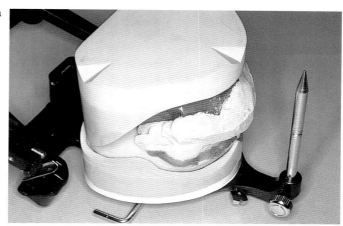

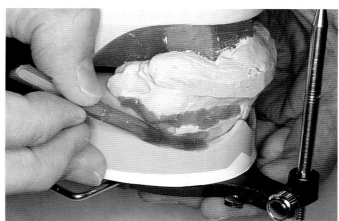

Fig. 9-241a, b   The lower cast temporarily attached to the articulator should be removed. The articulator should be placed upside down and the upper record base should be replaced on the upper cast. The lower record base should then be related to the upper record base using the interocclusal record and finally the lower cast should be seated in the lower record base. When the cast and record base, and the record base and plaster interocclusal record are joined together, they should be firmly attached to each other with sticky wax in turn, beginning with the upper cast and the upper record base.

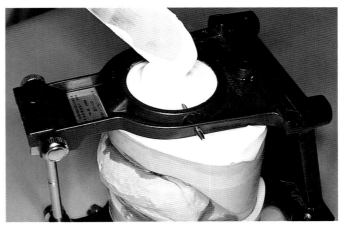

Fig. 9-242   A strip of vinyl tape should be wrapped around the lower cast. The cast should be mounted with stone that possesses a reduced setting expansion. If the upper and lower casts have not been securely joined and fixed using the interocclusal record and record bases, the recorded jaw relation will be spoiled during the mounting of the lower cast.

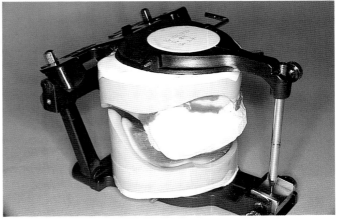

Fig. 9-243   The lower cast has been mounted using the plaster interocclusal record obtained in the centric occlusal position. In other words, the lower cast has finally been positioned on the articulator with the desired horizontal relation to the upper cast.

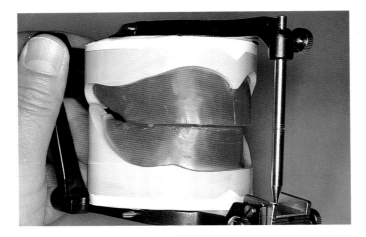

a

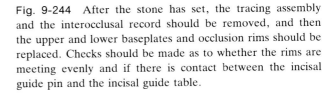

Fig. 9-244 After the stone has set, the tracing assembly and the interocclusal record should be removed, and then the upper and lower baseplates and occlusion rims should be replaced. Checks should be made as to whether the rims are meeting evenly and if there is contact between the incisal guide pin and the incisal guide table.

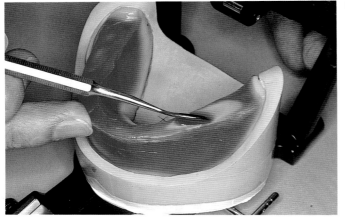

b

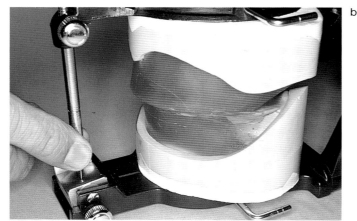

Fig. 9-245a, b In this case, there is a posterior premature contact and a small gap is found between the incisal guide pin and the incisal guide table. The surface of the upper rim should be smeared with vaseline, the surface of the lower rim should be softened using a similar technique to that used during the jaw registration and then the articulator should be closed. The rims meet evenly all the way around the arch.

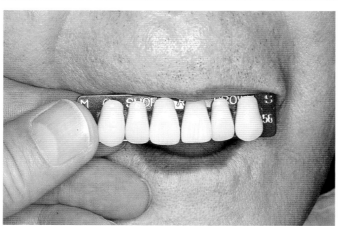

Fig. 9-246 The marks made on the upper rim at the corners of the mouth serve as a guide for selecting the size of the upper anterior teeth. When the shade and mold of the upper anterior teeth are being chosen, a better estimation of the chosen teeth can be gained by holding them in the mouth. At this time, the patient should be asked about his/her desires regarding the size, shape and shade of the teeth.

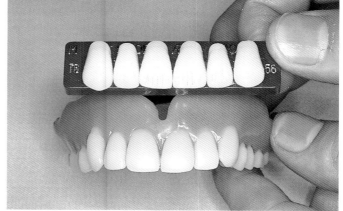

Fig. 9-247 If the patient wears dentures, tooth selection will be simplified by referring to their teeth. Simultaneously, the patient's comments about the teeth of the existing dentures should be asked.

a

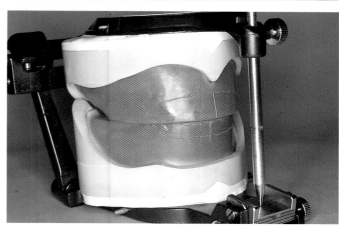

b

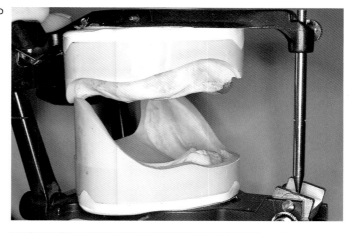

Fig. 9-248a, b Prior to the arrangement of the artificial teeth, the occlusion rims should be removed in turn and the orientation of the occlusal plane should be examined again by referring to the vertical relationship of the upper and lower ridges. In this case, the occlusal plane is situated in a well-balanced vertical position between the upper and lower ridges. If the occlusal plane is in a poorly balanced position, it should be adjusted based on the thinking that the occlusal plane divides the distance between the ridges in two. The amount of alveolar bone resorption should be considered when making the decision. If time is limited or the degree of adjustment is small, the desired inclination of the occlusal plane can be scored on the buccal surface of the rim which will serve as a guide for arranging the teeth.

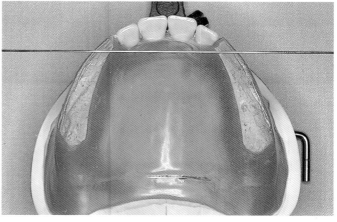

Fig. 9-249a The preliminary arrangement of the anterior teeth should be based on the standard positions of those teeth. The accurately carved occlusion rims serve as a guide for the arrangement of the anterior teeth. The central incisors should be set so that their labial surfaces are aligned with the labial surface of the wax rim.

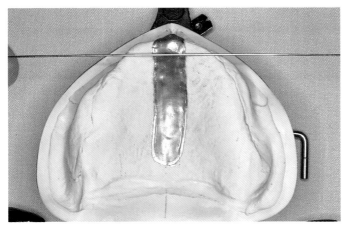

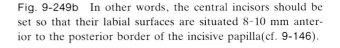

Fig. 9-249b   In other words, the central incisors should be set so that their labial surfaces are situated 8-10 mm anterior to the posterior border of the incisive papilla(cf. 9-146).

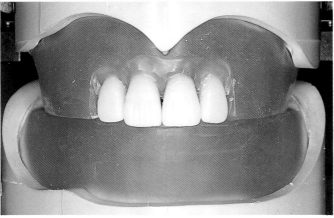

Fig. 9-250   The long axis of the central incisor should be approximately vertical. The incisal edge should be approximately 1 mm lower than the occlusal plane. The lateral incisor should be set slightly more lingual than the central incisor and moreover placed slightly inward at the neck. The incisal edge of the lateral incisor should touch the occlusal plane, and the axis should be inclined distally.

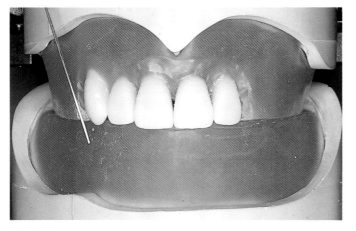

Fig. 9-251   The canine should be set more prominently than the other teeth and moreover, buccally at the neck. In this manner, the labial surface has a prominence at the neck which produces the effect that the labial surface is inclined out towards the neck.

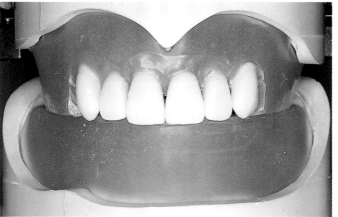

Fig. 9-252   As a result, the canine looks like a support. The distally inclined central and lateral incisors seem to be supported by the canine. If the canine does not appear to support the incisors, the anterior teeth will appear unstable.

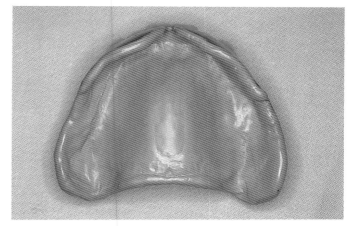

Fig. 9-253 If the upper anterior teeth have been set anteroposteriorly in the position occupied by the natural teeth by referring to the incisive papilla, when viewed from the basal surface of the upper trial denture base, the labial surfaces of the anterior teeth will be apparent. Also make certain that an imaginary transverse line extended between the upper canines crosses close to the posterior margin of the incisive papilla.

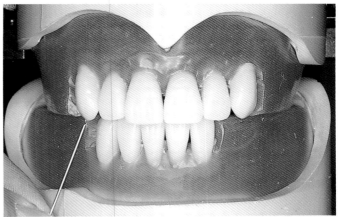

a

Fig. 9-254 The lower anterior teeth should be set anteroposteriorly according to the labial surface of the carved occlusion rim. However, the position of the residual ridge should be checked again and the artificial teeth should be placed as close as possible to the position occupied by the natural teeth by considering the amount of bone resorption. The edges of the anterior teeth should be aligned with the occlusal plane. The long axes of the central incisors are almost vertical, the long axes of the lateral incisors incline slightly distally at the neck, and the long axes of the canines incline still more distally at the neck. The canines look like firmly placed feet leading to a stable appearance of the anterior teeth.

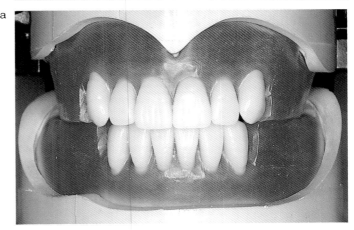

b

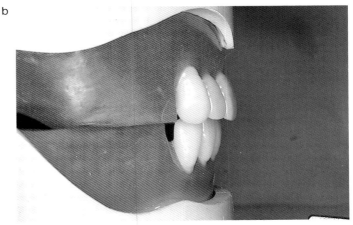

Fig. 9-255a, b A 1-1.5 mm vertical overlap has been provided. In order to avoid an impact between the opposing anterior teeth and an upward thrust in the anterior region due to the settling of dentures after insertion, the upper and lower anterior teeth should be arranged so as not to contact each other in the centric occlusal position, even though they were in contact in the natural dentition. By providing such a horizontal overlap, the incisal guide inclination is reduced and then the stability of the complete dentures will also be improved.

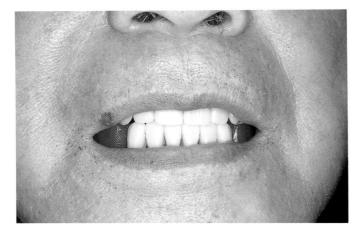

Fig. 9-256 When trying in the wax trial dentures, the dentist should check the labial fullness, the degree to which the upper and lower teeth are exposed, the midline, and the inclinations of teeth. They should be checked by referring to the overall balance of the face as well as the appearance around the mouth. Simultaneously, the desires and approval of the patient should be obtained. In order to make the patient keep the dentures in the mouth, it is essential to create the appearance that the patient desires. It is said that the dentist worries about only the retention and stability of the dentures, but the patient thinks that a good denture is one which looks good.

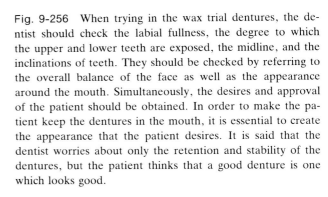

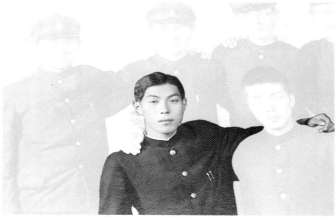

Fig. 9-257 A photograph of the patient with natural teeth can be most helpful during the try-in procedure for checking the arrangement of the anterior teeth. Even though the teeth are not apparent on the photograph, the appearance of the lower facial region when the teeth were present can be assessed.

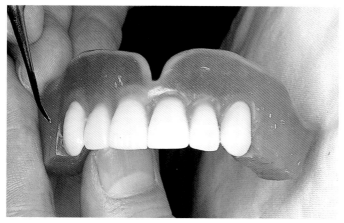

Fig. 9-258 As this patient has retired from work, a vigorous appearance should be avoided. So, in order to express the appearance of a gentle old man a softer expression of the canines has been created by reducing their prominence at the neck. However, if the distolabial portion of the canine can be seen when viewed from the front, the overall appearance will look inharmonious, so care must be taken when adjusting the canines.

a

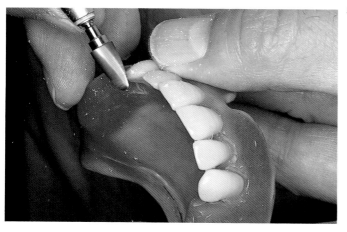

Fig. 9-259a, b The incisal edges of the natural anterior teeth wear with age. Concerning the artificial teeth, the tips of the canines are too pointed, causing an unnatural appearance. Therefore the incisal edges of the denture teeth should be ground to simulate the wear and tear that would have occurred at the patient's age.

b

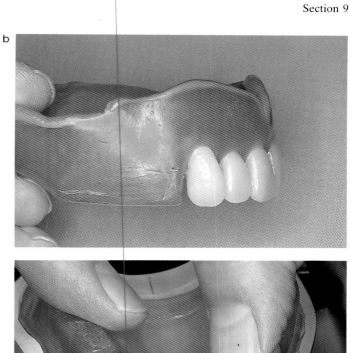

Fig. 9-260 Slightly rotating the mesial edges in and the distal edges out emphasizes the presence of the two central incisors, creating the appearance of youth.

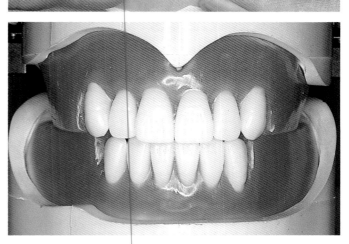

Fig. 9-261 After the teeth have been realigned, any excess wax around the necks of the teeth should be removed. At the try-in for the arrangement of the anterior teeth, it is essential to check the level of the gingival margins. If necessary, the positions of the upper canines may be readjusted after the arrangement of the molar teeth.

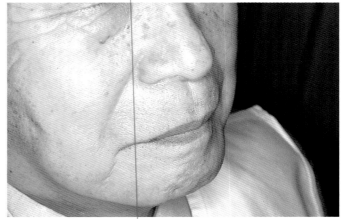

Fig. 9-262a Both trial dentures should be inserted after the positions of the anterior teeth have been adjusted. The anterior teeth provide adequate lip support, leading to a natural appearance.

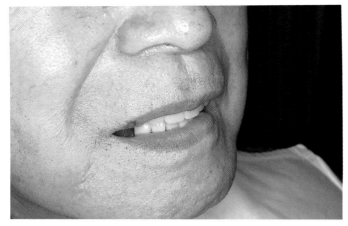

Fig. 9-262b Concerning the vertical positions of the anterior teeth, the upper and lower teeth should be evenly visible during speech or when smiling.

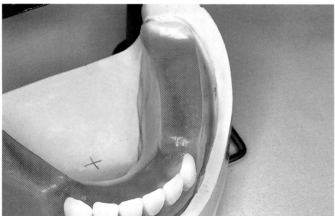

Fig. 9-263a The posterior teeth should be arranged in the center of the posterior denture-bearing area on the cast containing the external oblique ridge and mylohyoid ridge.

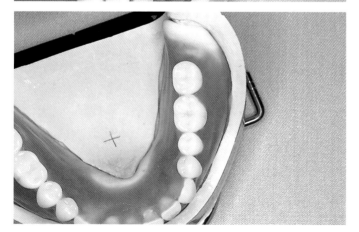

Fig. 9-263b Regarding the size of the posterior teeth, a small size should be used except in cases with markedly wide and favorable ridges. In this case, BioACE20° posterior teeth M28 (Shofu Co.) are used. The use of small sized teeth is essential to reduce the load on the supporting tissues and provide the desired shape for the polished surface. The dentist should not worry about the posterior slope of the lower ridge or should not eliminate one premolar tooth. The artificial teeth are much smaller than the natural teeth, so if there is not enough space for their arrangement, then the reasons for this must be investigated before proceeding. It may be that the anterior teeth have been arranged too far lingually.

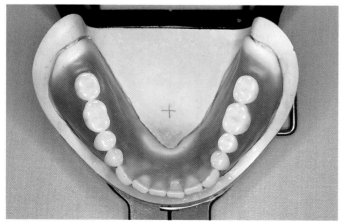

Fig. 9-263c A low cusp inclination should be chosen to minimize the lateral forces that will disturb the stability of the dentures.

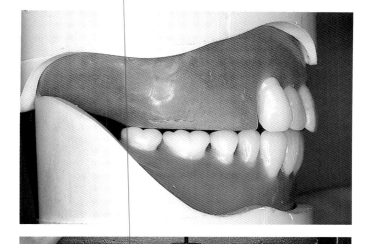

Fig. 9-264a   The level of the occlusal plane has been sufficiently examined using the wax rims. However, when arranging the posterior teeth, the occlusal plane may be slightly adjusted by referring to the lateral balance of the heights of the left and right posterior teeth.

Fig. 9-264b   In order to develop a balanced occlusion, the lower posterior teeth should be arranged along anteroposterior and lateral compensating curves, using the occlusal plane on the upper wax rim as a guide.

a

b

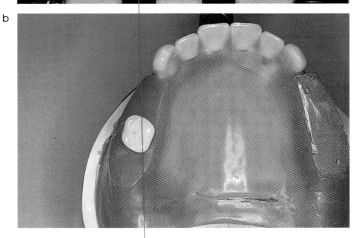

Fig. 9-265a, b   The upper posterior teeth should be arranged so as to approach the position occupied by the natural teeth by referring to the remnants of the lingual gingival margins, the cordlike elevation of mucosa situated near the crest of the residual ridge. The remnants move outwards according to the resorption of the residual ridge, so the posterior teeth should be arranged so as to sit partly on these remnants. Initially, the maxillary first molar should be placed in an approximately correct position, but slightly high.

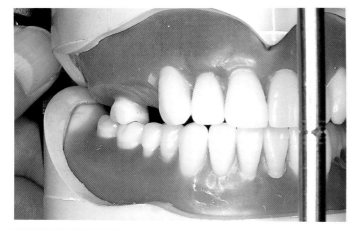

Fig. 9-266   The articulator should then be gently closed so that the opposing teeth push the maxillary first molar up to the desired level. While the articulator is closed, the maxillary first molar should be guided with the fingers to intercuspate with the opposing teeth. If the maxillary first molar is considerably displaced from its original position(cf. 9-265b), the opposing teeth should be removed and the upper and lower molar teeth should then be reset in a buccolingual position where they are in harmony with each other.

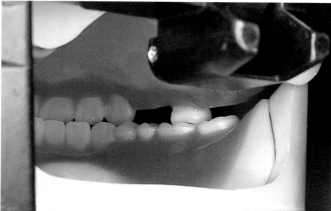

Fig. 9-267   From the lingual aspect, make certain that the mesiolingual cusp of the upper first molar is well seated in the central fossa of the lower first molar.

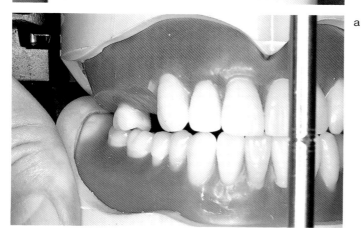

a

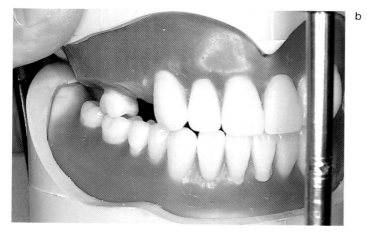

b

Fig. 9-268a, b   The articulator should be gently moved into lateral positions and the inclination of the maxillary first molar adjusted so as to eliminate any major interferences in working occlusion and balancing contact. The occlusal surfaces of the upper posterior teeth face outwards and those of the lower teeth face inwards. Final balancing of the teeth will be attained during the occlusal correction procedure after processing.

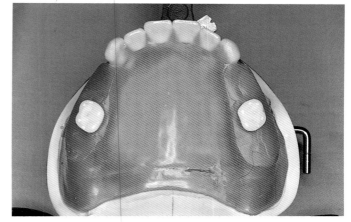

Fig. 9-269 Follow the same procedure in placing the maxillary first molar on the opposite side. The left and right upper first molars should be placed symmetrically.

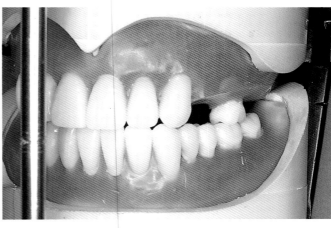

Fig. 9-270 After setting the left maxillary first molar to intercuspate with the opposing teeth, the relationships between the first molar and the opposing teeth in working occlusion and balancing contact should be checked. If necessary, the inclination of the upper maxillary first molar should be adjusted.

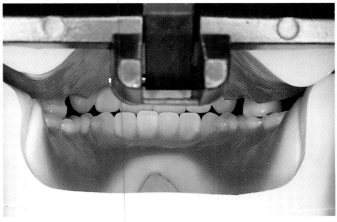

Fig. 9-271 Also from the lingual aspect, the interrelationship between the upper first molars and the lower first and second molars should be checked in working occlusion and balancing contact by moving the articulator laterally.

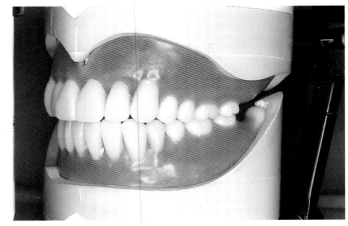

Fig. 9-272 The upper second premolar, first premolar and second molar should be set in turn, using a similar technique to that used for the upper first molars.

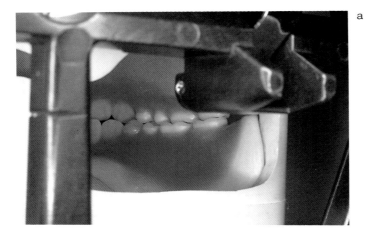

a

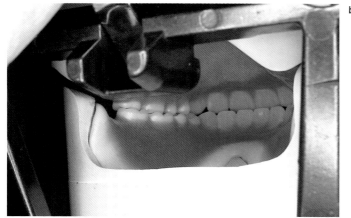

b

Fig. 9-273a, b There may be the possibility that the relationship between the upper and lower posterior teeth made in the centric occlusal position has been spoiled while adjusting the inclinations of the teeth in eccentric occlusion. So look from the lingual aspect to ensure that the upper posterior teeth remain in correct contact with the lower posterior teeth in the centric occlusal position.

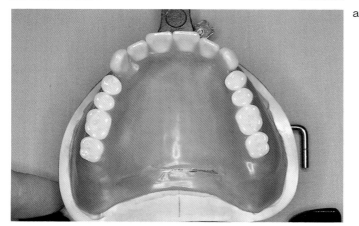

a

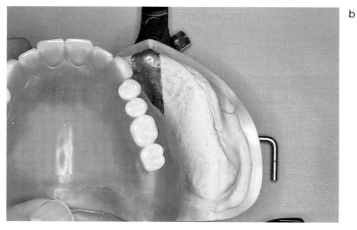

b

Fig. 9-274a, b An occlusal view of the maxillary wax denture after the arrangement of the posterior teeth. The artificial posterior teeth have not been placed on the so-called alveolar crest, but rather, have been arranged in the position occupied by the natural teeth by referring to the remnants of the lingual gingival margins. As a result, we can see the rounded arch of the artificial teeth without any inward curves in the premolar regions.

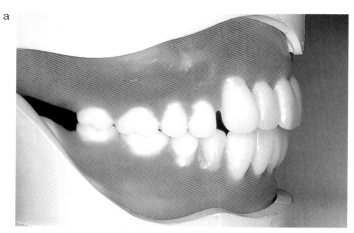

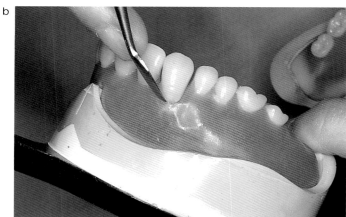

Fig. 9-275a, b   In this case, a space has developed between the maxillary canine and premolar after the arrangement of the posterior teeth, so the long axis of the maxillary canine must be inclined somewhat distally at the neck. If the space is narrower than 1 mm, it is not necessary to adjust the canine.

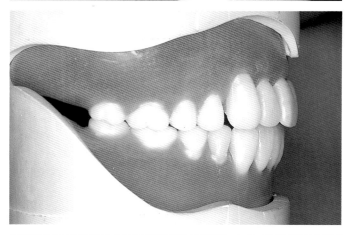

Fig. 9-276   By moving the canine slightly inward while inclining it distally, the width of the space has been reduced. The shifted canine must be rechecked for esthetics in the mouth at the try-in appointment for checking the arrangement of the posterior teeth.

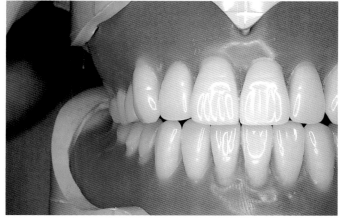

Fig. 9-277   The inclination of the buccal surface of the maxillary first premolar is not aligned with that of the maxillary canine and thus continuity between the anterior teeth and the posterior teeth is broken, leading to a poor appearance.

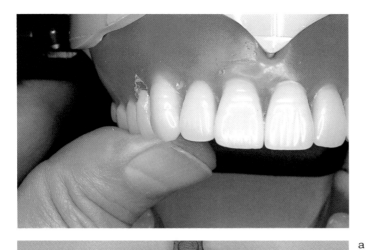

Fig. 9-278 The first premolar should be moved buccally at the neck so that the inclination of its buccal surface is aligned with that of the canine. The first premolar links the anterior teeth and posterior teeth, so the esthetic effect of the first premolar must not be forgotten. It is not a problem if the lingual cusp of the premolar does not occlude with the lower tooth due to this adjustment.

a

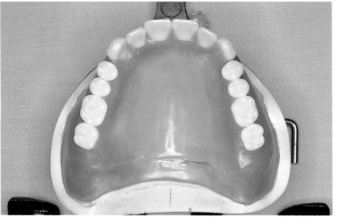

b

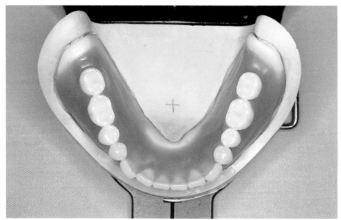

Fig. 9-279a, b Occlusal views of the completed tooth arrangement. By placing the artificial teeth in the position occupied by the natural teeth, a large tongue space has been obtained. After a rough waxing, the try-in procedure for checking the arrangement of the posterior teeth should be performed. At this try-in appointment, the occlusion can be checked roughly, but the occlusal contacts and phonetics can not be checked adequately because the wax dentures move easily. Tests for denture retention and stability are out of the question.

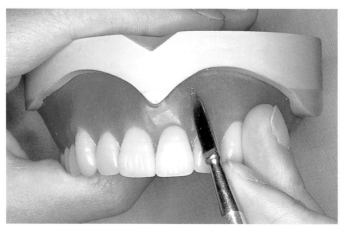

Fig. 9-280 Creating prominences is not necessary in the regions which correspond to the roots of the anterior teeth. However, a slight eminence should be formed all over the flange, starting from the necks and eventually blending into the denture border.

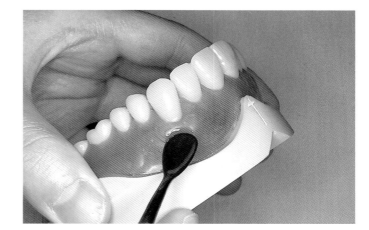

Fig. 9-281 Above the canine tooth, a large eminence should be produced for lip support by referring to the appearance.

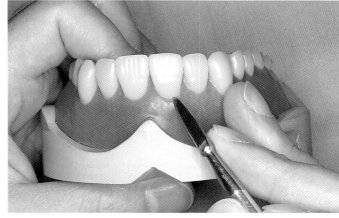

Fig. 9-282 In the dentate person, the gingival margin recedes with aging. The height of the gingival margins of the denture depends on age, and so they should be formed so that at least the finish lines on the necks of the artificial teeth can be seen in a patient who is older than sixty years. The gingival margins of the upper lateral incisors should be situated lower than the other upper anterior teeth. The interdental papilla of the denture should be formed deep and low.

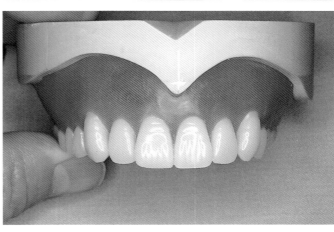

Fig. 9-283 If the upper anterior teeth have been appropriately set vertically, only a small portion of the gingiva is visible even when smiling. Therefore it is not necessary to develop root prominences in the regions which correspond to the roots. The appearance of the neck regions which are visible when smiling is important.

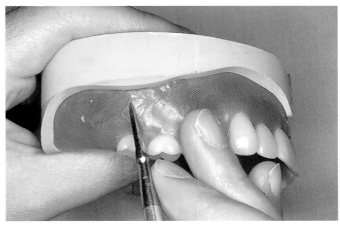

Fig. 9-284 Root prominences in the posterior region should not be provided because they cause a strange sensation in the patient's mouth, and will lead to the accumulation of food. The buccal surface from the necks to the denture border should be made convex.

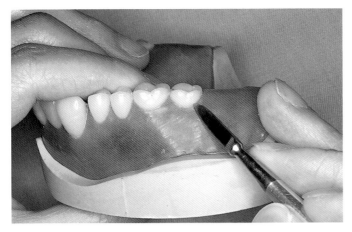

Fig. 9-285 The interdental papilla should be carved high and sharply.

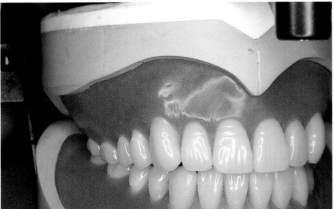

Fig. 9-286 The gingival margin of the first premolar should be carved so as to avoid a sudden step down from the canine to the premolar. A marked difference between the levels of the margins of these two teeth will spoil the appearance of the dentures. A long premolar tooth should be used to raise the level of its gingival margin.

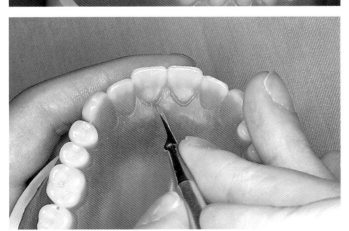

Fig. 9-287 The lingual surface should be contoured to simulate the normal palate. In order to attain clear 'S' sounds, a reverse curve should be reproduced in the region of the incisive papilla.

a

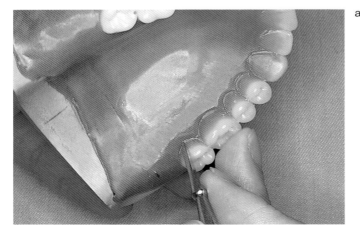

Fig. 9-288a, b The posterior palatal alveolar area should also be slightly thickened to allow normal tongue contact during speech(Fig. b, arrow). However, if the level of the gingival margins of the artificial teeth has been carved lower, the adjacent thickened area will be lowered (Fig. b, dotted line). This will make speech awkward and indistinct.

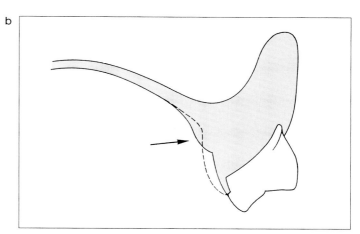

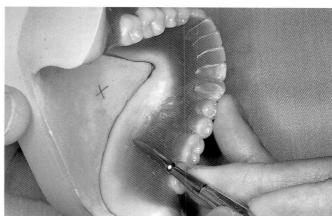

Fig. 9-289 The lingual surface from the necks of the teeth to the periphery in the lower posterior region should be contoured to produce a concave form. Care should be taken not to extend the concavity under the lingual surface of the teeth, otherwise the tongue will slip into the undercut and dislodge the denture.

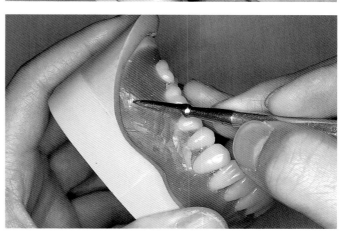

Fig. 9-290 The buccal surface should be contoured slightly convex or straight.

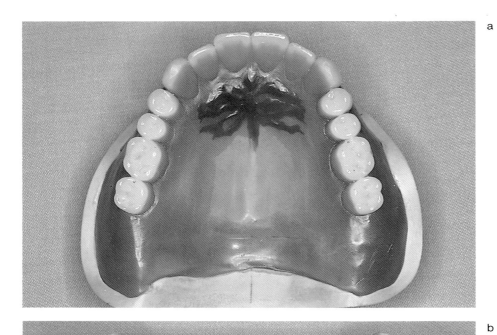

a

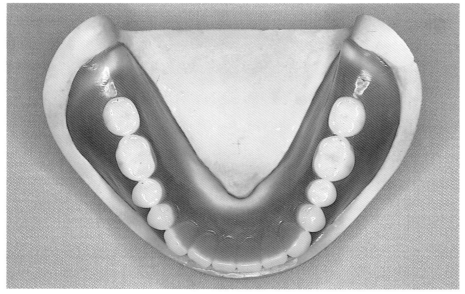

b

c

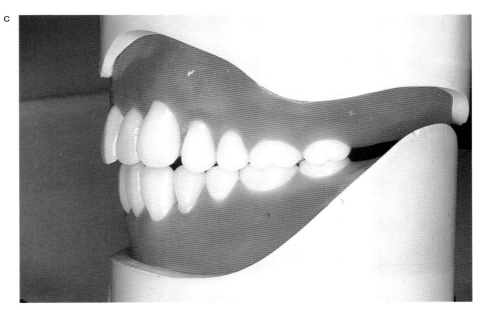

d

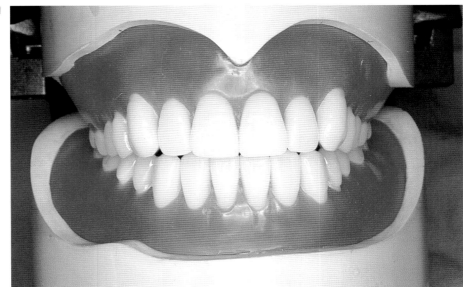

e

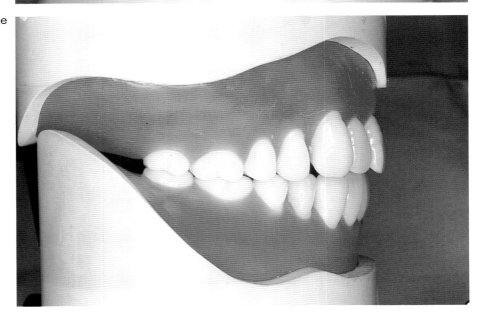

Fig. 9-291a ～ e The upper and lower waxed-up dentures.

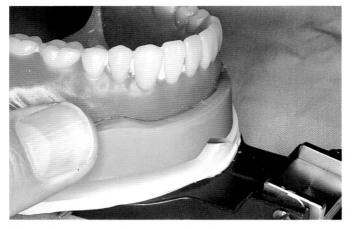

Fig. 9-292   After the denture has been cured, the denture and cast should be removed from the flask as one unit. The cast with the processed denture should be remounted on the articulator using the V-shaped notches.

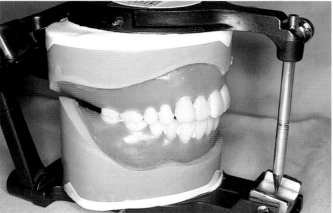

Fig. 9-293   Make certain that the cast and mounting stone fit together accurately. The cast should then be joined to the mounting stone in the frame of the articulator by sticking a strip of vinyl tape along the junction.

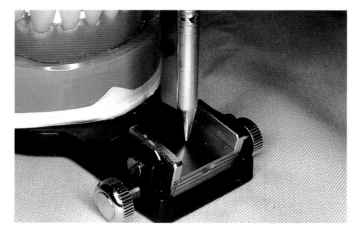

Fig. 9-294   The incisal guide pin does not contact the incisal guide table due to changes in occlusion that have occurred during processing. These occlusal errors should be eliminated by appropriately grinding the occlusal surfaces of the denture teeth. Furthermore, the occlusal surfaces should be ground into harmony with the jaw movements. In this case, the selective grinding to obtain a balanced occlusion is performed to ensure that any interferences are not built into the occlusion.

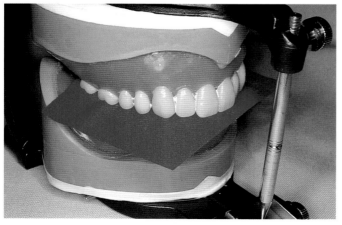

Fig. 9-295   Place articulating paper between the teeth, and gently tap the teeth together.

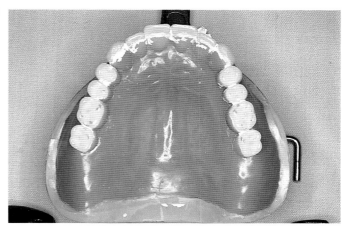

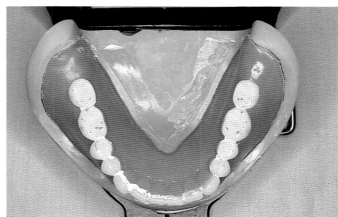

Fig. 9-296a, b   There are a few occlusal contacts between the dentures in the centric occlusal position.

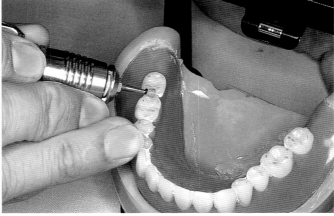

Fig. 9-297   Premature contacts should be corrected with small stones. Grinding should be done in the fossae and not on the cusp tips, except in cases where the cusps are high in both the centric occlusal position and eccentric positions. This marking and grinding procedure should be repeated until all the teeth have even contact in the centric occlusal position.

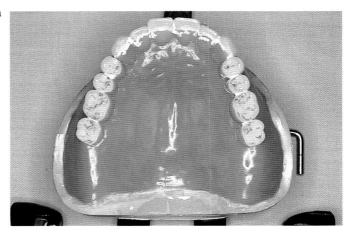

Fig. 9-298a, b   The adjustment in the centric occlusal position should be stopped when widespread contacts are produced.

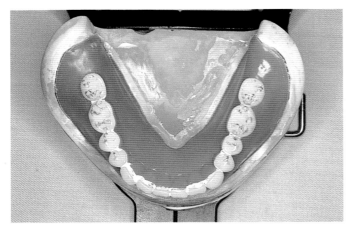

b

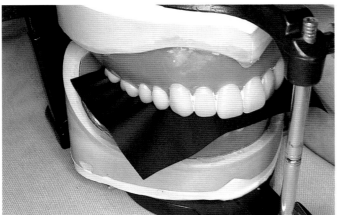

Fig. 9-299 Articulating paper should be placed over the teeth on both sides, and the articulator should be moved into one of the lateral positions. The contacts will be marked on both sides for the same lateral movement. Articulating paper of a different color should be used to distinguish the contacts marked in eccentric positions from those marked in the centric occlusal position.

a

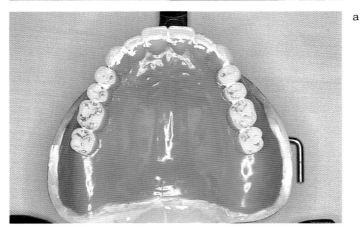

b

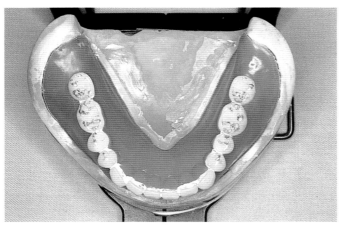

Fig. 9-300a, b Blue articulating paper has been used to locate the deflective occlusal contacts in right lateral occlusion. Examine the resulting pattern on the working and balancing sides.

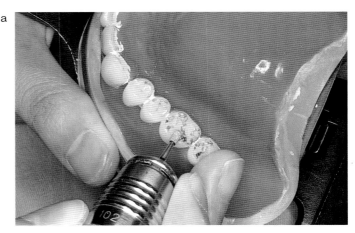

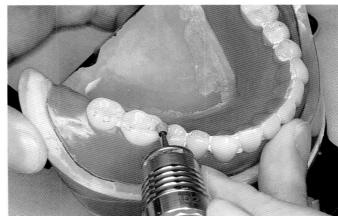

Fig. 9-301a, b Eliminate deflective contacts by grinding the lingual inclines of the upper buccal cusps and the buccal inclines of the lower lingual cusps on the working side. This is the so-called BULL rule. The lingual cusps of the upper teeth and the buccal cusps of the lower teeth should not be ground, or the occlusal vertical dimension will be decreased. On the balancing side, mainly the lingual inclines of the lower buccal cusps should be ground for the adjustment.

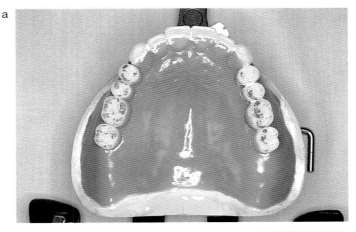

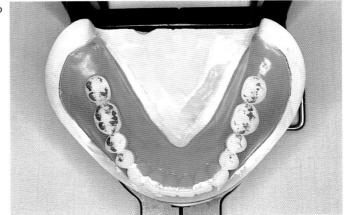

Fig. 9-302a, b The marking and grinding procedure should be repeated for the right lateral movement until the markings made by the movements indicate uniform contacts on the working and balancing sides.

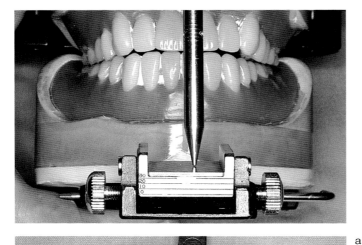

a

Fig. 9-303 When the selective grinding in lateral occlusion has almost been completed, the incisal guide pin usually stays in contact with the incisal guide table during lateral excursions.

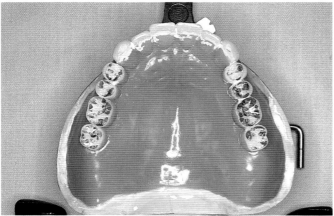

b

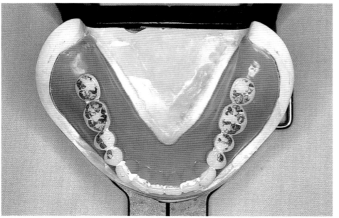

Fig. 9-304a, b The same procedure should be performed in left lateral and protrusive movements. After completing the selective grinding, markings made by movements in all directions should show uniform contacts. The red articulating paper marks show contacts made in the centric occlusal position and the blue marks show contacts made during lateral and protrusive movements.

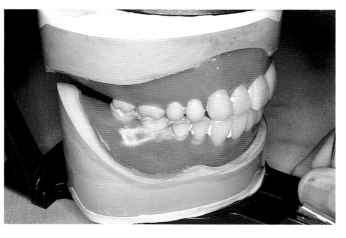

Fig. 9-305 Minute irregularities should be smoothed by carborundum paste in gliding movements of the articulator.

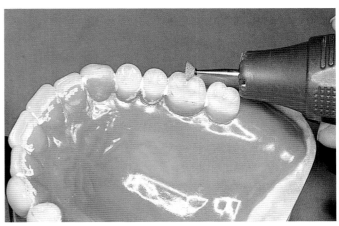

Fig. 9-306 The fossae and fissures may have been removed to a certain extent by the grinding procedure and thus the area of contact between the occlusal surfaces unnecessarily increased, leading to poor masticatory efficiency. Therefore the fissures should be deepened with a small stone to ensure the food exits during function properly.

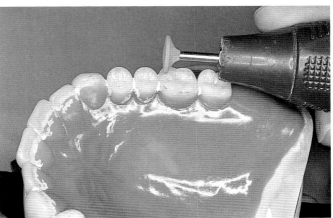

Fig. 9-307 Roughened surfaces should be smoothed with a silicon polishing point.

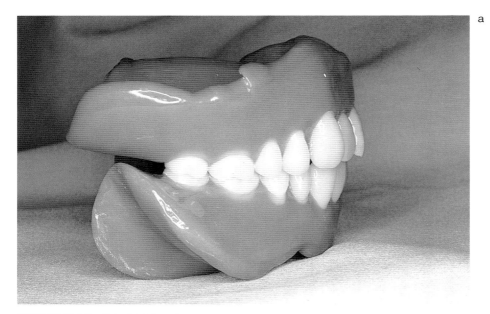

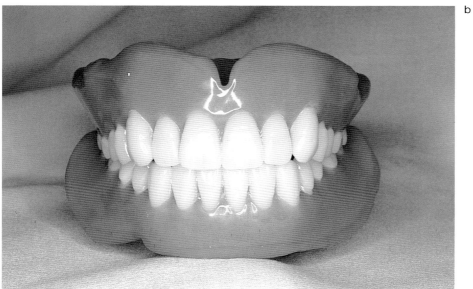

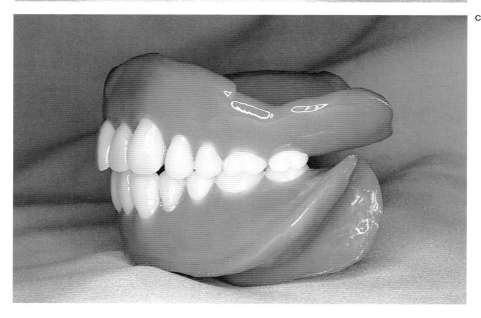

Fig. 9-308a～k　Dentures having a well-balanced form function sufficiently well.

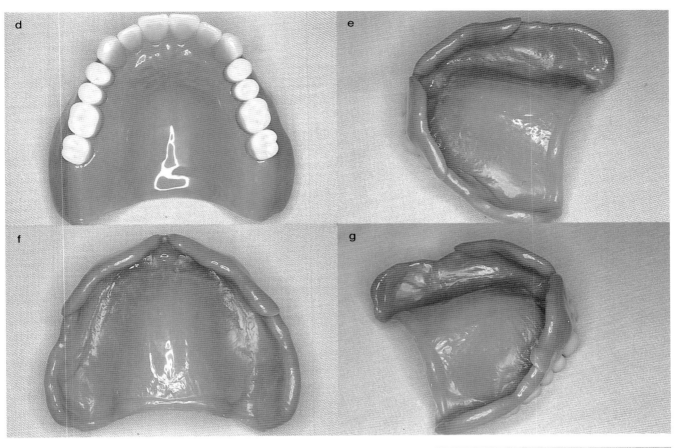

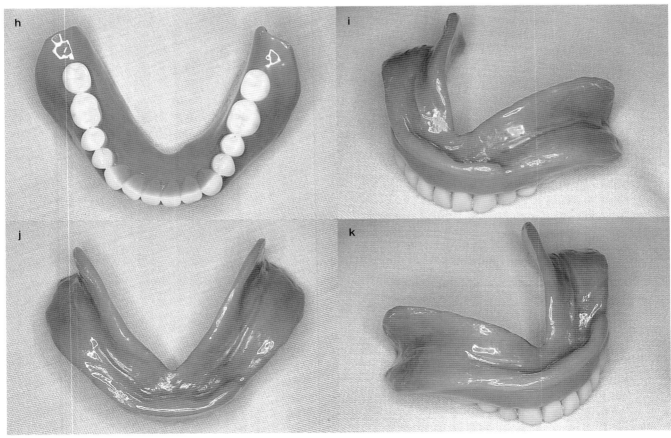

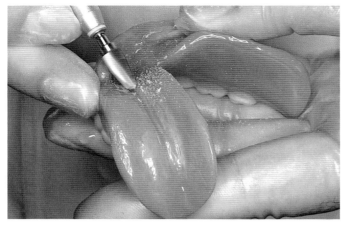

Fig. 9-309 Prior to inserting the completed dentures, the fitting surfaces should be carefully inspected by palpation and any sharp projections should be ground away. The pain patients experience just after inserting new dentures may lead them to lose confidence in the dentures. This will make acceptance of the new dentures difficult.

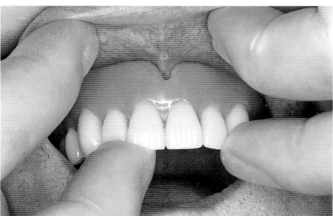

Fig. 9-310 At first, insert the maxillary denture into the mouth and make certain that the length of the denture border is properly extended. The frenum may have been displaced while making the impression, so the frenal area should be carefully checked.

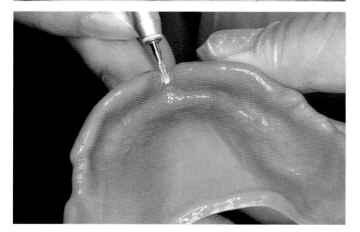

Fig. 9-311 In this case, the labial frenum is slightly displaced by the notched border of the denture, so the notch should be slightly deepened and widened vertically with a large fissure bur. Also bevel the inner margin of the notch according to the form of the frenum.

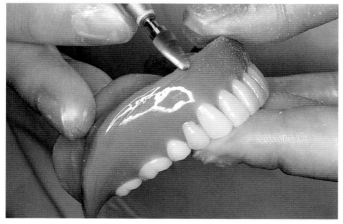

Fig. 9-312 The denture border of the mandibular denture should be checked in the mouth, and if necessary, it should be adjusted. In the mentalis muscle area and retromolar pad area, the impression tends to be overextended, so the examination should be carefully performed.

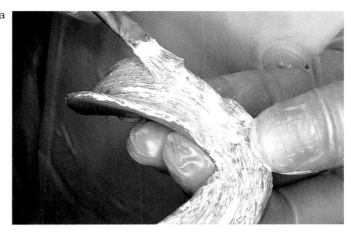

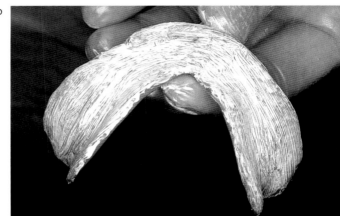

Fig. 9-313a, b   Pressure indicating paste is used to detect areas on the denture base which exert excessive pressure on the residual ridge. A thin layer of paste should be painted on the fitting surface of the denture so that the brush marks are visible.

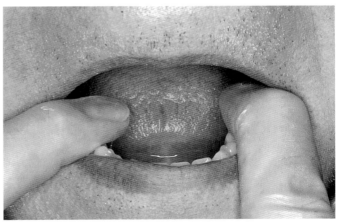

Fig. 9-314   The denture should be carefully placed on the residual ridge and heavy pressure should be applied on the occlusal surface of the teeth with the fingers. The location of pressure spots in the denture base that displace soft tissue can then be determined. By eliminating the pressure spots appropriately, the dentures will not trouble the patient when an occlusal force is applied. In cases where little pressure was applied when the impression was made, this procedure is particularly important.

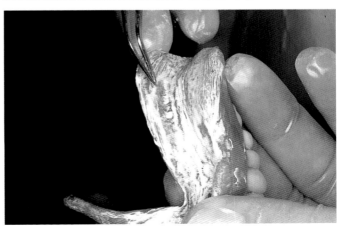

Fig. 9-315   An area where the paste is very thin or completely displaced indicates pressure spots.

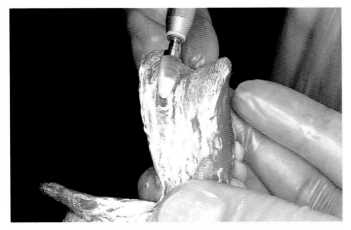

Fig. 9-316 This lower denture displays a point of pressure on the mylohyoid ridge. This pressure spot should be relieved with a bur.

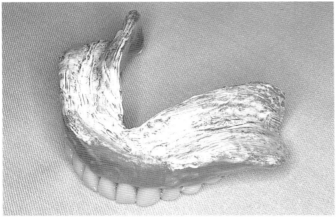

Fig. 9-317 This recording and trimming should be repeated until the surface of the denture base does not show through the paste and the paste layer is reasonably even. The resilience of the soft tissue varies depending on the area, so a completely even layer of the paste can not expected.

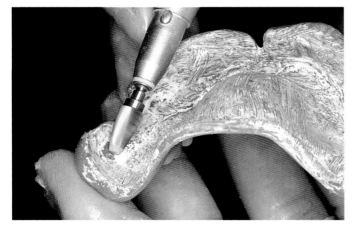

Fig. 9-318 Follow the same procedure for detecting and relieving pressure spots from the maxillary denture base. The paste layer may be displaced due to brushing against the residual ridge on insertion and removal of the denture, so it should be carefully determined as to whether the areas with the displaced paste are pressure areas or the result of accidental contact during insertion and removal.

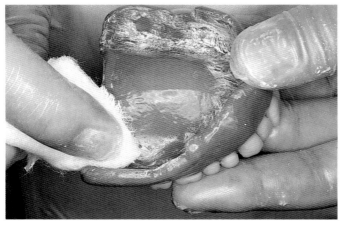

Fig. 9-319 Pressure indicating paste should be wiped off with cotton using firm, uni-directional strokes, not in a back and forth motion. Even if small projections disappear on the fitting surface of denture base, they can be easily found because cotton fibers will be caught on the spikes.

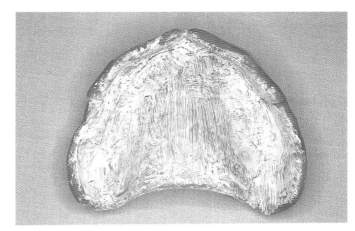

Fig. 9-320 A fairly even paste record. No more adjustments are necessary.

a

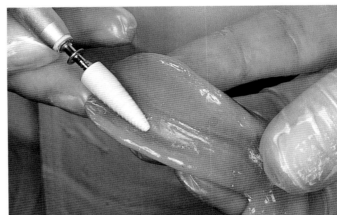

b

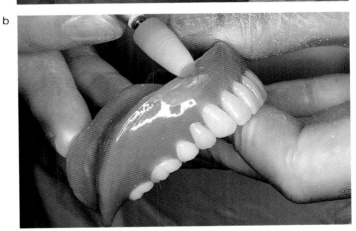

Fig. 9-321a, b Areas roughened during the adjustment of the basal surface should be smoothed with a sandpaper cone and polished with a silicone point for the resin base.

Fig. 9-322 After adjusting the basal surface, refinement of the occlusion should be carried out at the chairside. Prior to occlusal adjustment, cotton rolls should be placed on both sides between the upper and lower posterior teeth. The patient should be instructed to bite them for about ten minutes. In this manner the underlying tissue will become accustomed to the fit of the new dentures. When biting the cotton rolls, if the patient complains of some irritation of the tissues, the soreness could not have resulted from errors in occlusion because the patient is not allowed to close on the teeth. Therefore adjustment of the fitting surface should be performed again.

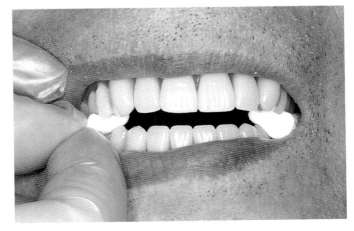

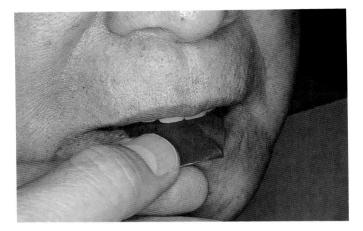

Fig. 9-323 In denture fabrication, small unavoidable errors occur during each procedure, and the accumulation of these errors leads to problems with the occlusion when new dentures are first inserted. Therefore occlusal adjustment is always necessary when inserting new dentures. As a first step, occlusal contacts between the dentures in the centric occlusal position should be checked using thin articulating paper.

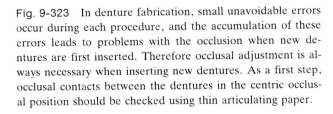

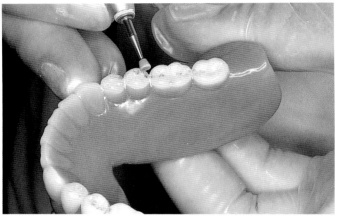

Fig. 9-324 The heavy contacts in the centric occlusal position should be corrected by grinding the fossae and inclines of the cusps.

a

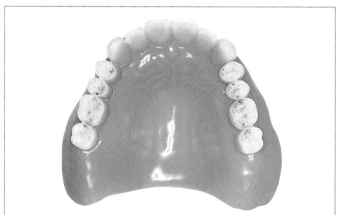

b

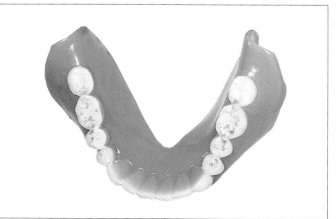

Fig. 9-325a, b These procedures should be repeated until the posterior teeth have almost even occlusal contacts in the centric occlusal position.

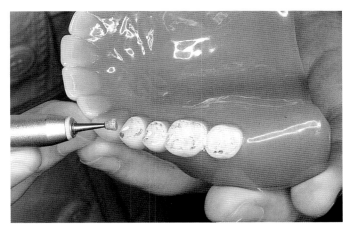

Fig. 9-326 If interferences are found when the jaw is moved to the left and right, or protruded, they should be eliminated in the same manner as was used during the selective grinding on the articulator.

a

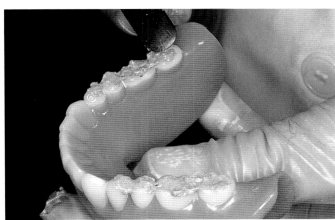

b

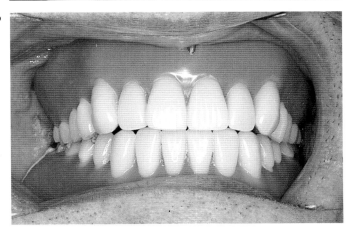

Fig. 9-327a, b   An even layer of carborundum paste should be placed on the occlusal surface of the lower posterior teeth. The patient should be asked to slowly move the jaw to the left and right, and anteroposteriorly. By grinding with carborundum paste in the mouth, the facets of the upper and lower teeth, which are in harmony with the patient's mandibular movements, can be established. Simultaneously the cuspal inclines may be reduced and some occlusal freedom can be produced. In elderly patients, the mandibular joints are loose and the muscles of mastication function poorly. Therefore even though the correct centric occlusal position has been obtained, the position is unstable, so providing some occlusal freedom is essential.

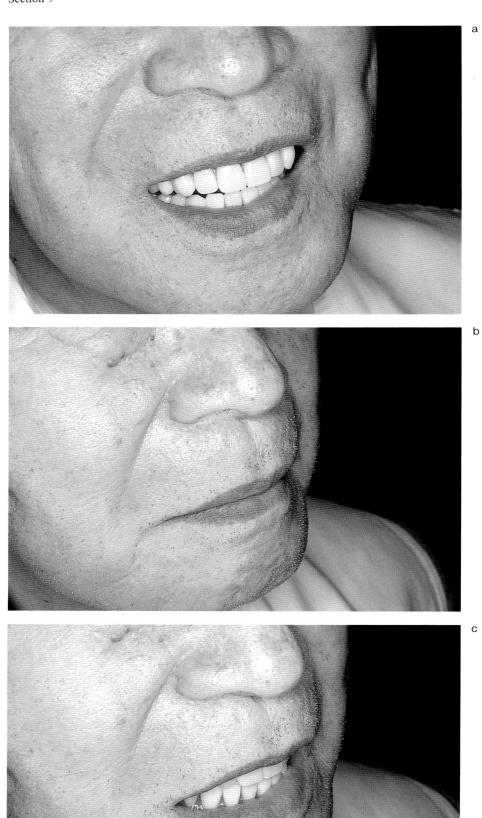

Fig. 9-328a ～ c Appearance with new dentures.

Appendix

Application of soft denture lining materials

Application of soft denture lining materials

Occasionally, even though the denture borders are appropriately extended, the arrangement of the artificial teeth and the occlusion are satisfactory, and also the stability and retention of the denture are good, pain occurs under the denture during mastication, which is difficult to relieve.

In the case of an extremely resorbed residual ridge, the overlying mucosa decreases in thickness according to the resorption. As the shock-absorbing effect of the mucosa is diminished and masticatory impact forces are directly transmitted to the underlying tissues, the burden on the residual ridge is increased. In addition, lesions may be created and generalized irritation or soreness is seen on the basal seat because the thin mucosa is pinched between the hard denture base and the nonresilient bony support during mastication. In such a case with thin mucosa, advanced measures are necessary. In other words, it is necessary to line the inner surface of the denture base with a soft material similar to the mucosa in order to compensate for the lost thickness and viscoelasticity of the mucosa. The pain is relieved by reducing the impact force during mastication and dispersing the masticatory force widely over the alveolar ridge to give a cushioning effect. The material used for this lining is called a "soft lining material"(Fig.A-1).

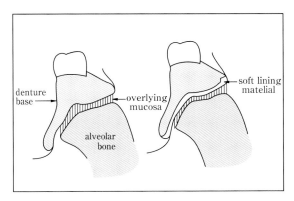

Fig. A-1 The lost thickness and viscoelasticity of the mucosa is compensated for by using a soft lining material.

1. Soft lining materials

The current soft lining materials are grouped into acrylic, silicone and fluorinated resins and recently an olefinic material has been developed.

1) Acrylic soft lining materials

These are plasticized self-curing or heat-curing acrylic resins. By adding a plasticizer, the resins can be rendered elastomeric. Strong adhesion of these liners to the acrylic resin denture base can be expected because of their composition.

However, the added plasticizer will gradually diffuse onto the surface of the resin and will be leached out by the saliva, resulting in a liner that will gradually harden[41]. Also, there is a problem of bacterial contamination which may be due to the roughness of the surface or water absorption of the material[42]. For example:

  Coe-soft(Coe), Soften(Kamemizu)······Direct method
  Super-soft(Coe)······Indirect method

2) Silicone soft lining materials

These possess the characteristics of an elastomer by mixing the silicone base and catalyst as with silicone rubber impression materials. The materials are chemically stable and thus the elasticity can be maintained, but as they do not directly adhere to acrylic resin, an adhesive is necessary. The bond strength of current adhesives has been improved, but is not yet sufficient. Therefore the bond must be strengthened by changing the lining form(See P. 244). After the surface of the lining material is trimmed for adjustments, the surface cannot be polished properly, so the roughened surface will be contaminated with food debris. In addition, as the silicone rubber is porous, food debris which stagnates inside the pores enhances the growth of fungi such as *Candida albicans*, leading to the formation of fungal colonies[43]. For example:

  Mollosil(DETAX), Evatouch(Neo)······Direct method
  Moloplast-B(DETAX)······Indirect method

3) Fluorinated soft lining material

This possesses excellent viscoelastic properties. It adheres well to the denture base resin because the fluorinated copolymer strongly bonds physically to acrylic resin[44]. The lining technique is easy, but if quick curing denture base resins are used, roughness or voids will occur on the surface of the lining material after polymerization. Contamination due to fungal colonies of *Candida albicans* etc. is minimal, but as plaque is observed on the liner after long term usage, the denture should sometimes be cleaned by denture cleansers for hygiene maintenance.

  Kurepeet Dough(Kureha)······Indirect method

4) Olefinic soft lining material

This possesses good elastic properties and chemical stability. However, special apparatus for lining is necessary and the lining procedure is complicated. As with silicone materials, an adhesive is necessary. Initially, the bond strength of the adhesive used for this method was not strong, but as the bonding method has improved, the bond strength has increased.

Water absorption is minimal, but as the liner tends to become discolored by food, a coating agent is indispensable to prevent such discoloration[45].

Molteno(Molten)⋯⋯Indirect method

These materials can be divided according to lining method; direct or indirect. Some materials can be used in both methods. In the direct method, an impression is made with a lining material applied to the tissue surface of the denture and then it is allowed to cure in the mouth. The procedure is somewhat simple and as it is done directly in the mouth, there is less likelihood of making errors. However, it tends to be contaminated by saliva etc. and as it is difficult to control the lining form, the required lining thickness cannot easily be obtained. Also, an overall even thickness of the lining is impossible to obtain. In addition, in some materials, the irritating monomers and the heat of polymerization may produce a disagreeable sensation on the mucosa. The physical properties of these materials obtained by the direct method are worse

Soft liners and viscoelasticity

Soft lining materials are usually termed a resilient liner. However, they should not have resiliency in the strict sense of the word. If the liner were truly resilient, the denture might tend to bounce away from the residual ridge with each application and release of masticatory force. In order that the soft liner functions as a shock absorber to ease masticatory loads, it is essential that the liner has the same viscoelasticity as the mucosa(Fig. 1). A slow recovery following deformation due to occlusal loading is more desirable than recovery that is instantaneously elastic[41,46].

From this point of view, the silicone and olefinic liners possess a rubber-like elasticity and the acrylic and fluorinated liners possess viscoelastic properties[47](Fig. 2). The current soft liners are mainly resilient, and even the viscoelastic types do not exhibit proper viscoelastic properties. The acrylic soft liners have a cushioning effect just after lining, but they tend to gradually harden. Fluorinated resin can not be considered to have the same viscoelasticity as the mucosa.

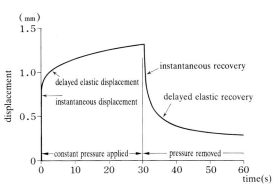

Fig. 1 The behavior of the mucosa under load and after load release[45].

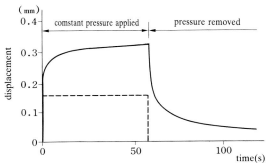

Fig. 2 The behavior of soft liners under load and after load release.(solid line: viscoelastic liner, dotted line: resilient liner).

than those of the indirect method. Therefore, the direct method should be performed only for temporary use or for a patient whose ability to visit the clinic is limited.

On the other hand, in the indirect method, the lining procedure is performed in the laboratory after impression making. One step is added, but the chairside time is decreased. In addition, each step can be checked, so the form and thickness of the lining material can be controlled.

Tissue conditioners

Tissue conditioners such as Hydro-Cast(Kay-See Dental), Visco-gel(Amalgamated Dental), Fitt(Kerr), Soft Liner(GC) and Comfort(Coe) that are used for conditioning the abused mucosa are also generally termed resilient liners. The composition of the powdered polymer is a poly(ethyl methacrylate), or one of its co-polymers and the liquid monomer is an aromatic ester in an alcohol solvent. By mixing them together a plastic gel is formed[41].

As the tissue conditioners can maintain their plasticity for just a short time, the mucosa distorted by an ill-fitting denture will recover after the denture is relined with them. They are also viscoelastic, so they can relieve pain during occlusion because of their cushioning effect. However, as they are soft materials of an unstable polymer, they absorb water and swell in the mouth, the effective compositions such as alcohol are leached out and thus the viscoelasticity will be lost in a short time. Therefore, if they are used for a long time, they may become hard and contaminated, which will further irritate the mucosa. Tissue conditioners are materials which are used temporarily for conditioning the mucosa and their purpose is quite different from that of soft liners and these two materials should be distinguished.

2. Indications

When using soft liners, it is important to examine each case as to whether or not a soft liner is really needed. Even though impression making or jaw registration is somewhat inadequate, if the errors are within the limits where they can be compensated for by the cushioning effect of the liner, the errors may become negligible. Soft liners should be effectively used only after mastering the techniques of impression making, jaw registration, etc. It would not be the right course to compensate for these errors just by using these materials. Stresses due to errors may lead to other problems.

The indications are as follows:

1) A case in which pain occurs during mastication because of

the thin overlying mucosa which has been caused by severe resorption of the alveolar bone.

2) A case in which pain occurs during mastication because of irregularly resorbed or sharpened alveolar bone.

3) A case with severe undercuts of the alveolar bone.

4) A case with a residual ridge which is unable to support the occlusal force adequately.

5) Obturators for maxillofacial prostheses.

It has also been reported that with the use of soft liners, as the occlusal force is evenly dispersed all over the residual ridge, it provides stimulation to the ridge leading to the reproduction of bone tissue[48]. The soft lining materials have also been reported to improve the retention and stability of the denture, and comfort of the patient[49]. In particular, there is no contraindication, but for a case where the overlying mucosa is quite thick and possesses the cushioning effect, the soft liner should not be used because it is beyond the indications for their use.

— How to evaluate a case requiring a soft liner —

When pain occurs during mastication with the existing dentures, one should firstly examine their form and fit, or the occlusion which may frequently be the cause of the pain. If errors are found, they should be corrected first. Only when the pain can not be relieved with these corrections, should one decide to use a soft liner. Those dentists who are not familiar with soft liners should firstly reline the denture base with a tissue conditioner and use it as a temporary soft liner for 1-2 months. From the result of using a tissue conditioner, it can almost be determined if the problem can be solved with a soft liner or not. If one determines the thickness or lining area of the tissue conditioner by the amount of removed resin from the inner surface of the denture base, it can become a good guide for the thickness and lining area of the soft liner. If a coating agent for tissue conditioners(Kregard, Kureha) is applied to the surface of the tissue conditioner, the durability of the conditioner will be greatly improved, leading to a denture that could be used for 1-2 months without changing the tissue conditioner[50,51] (Fig. A-2, 3). Kregard was developed by the author's research group.

Kregard

This is an ethyl acetate solution containing a fluorinated soft resin. It is applied to the surface of the tissue conditioner leaving the surface coated by a thin film of the fluorinated resin after the solvent has evaporated. Due to the characteristics of the fluorinated copolymer, the effective compo-

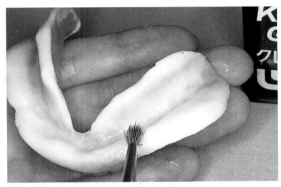

Fig. A-2 The longevity of a tissue conditioner will be greatly extended by covering the surface with the fluorinated coating agent(Kregard).

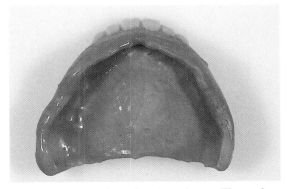

Fig. A-3 Clincal view after 2 weeks use.The surface treated with the fluorinated coating(left) has a shiny and smooth appearance, but the untreated half(right) has become irregular and roughened.

Table 1 Water sorption of tissue conditioners treated with the fluorinated coating agent(after immersion in 37°C water for 21 days).

Tissue Conditioners	Coating layers		
	No applications	One layer	Two layers
A	1.2	0.6	0.1
B	1.4	0.3	0.1
C	2.0	0.8	0.5
D	1.6	0.5	0.3
E	0.9	0.2	0.1

A. Hydro-cast,   B. Visco-gel,   C. Fitt,   unit : mg / cm^2
D. Soft Liner,   E. Coe-comfort

Table 2 Abrasion resistance of tissue conditioners treated with the fluorinated coating agent(load 166g/cm^2, stroke width 100 mm).

Number of Strokes	Tissue conditioner (A) Coating layers			Tissue conditioner (B) Coating layers		
	no	one	two	no	one	two
0	15	22	29	19	26	40
1000	10	20	23	12	26	35
3000	6	16	19	10	22	26

unit : gross values(%)

nents of the tissue conditioner will not be leached out and also excellent water resistance will be provided, thus the viscoelasticity of the conditioner will last longer. In addition, by coating the surface of the conditioner, it will become smoother and its abrasion resistance will also be improved. Therefore, it becomes possible to clean the surface of the liner adequately and thus contamination will be greatly reduced(Table 1, 2).

3. Clinical case

A case of severe alveolar ridge resorption with thin covering mucosa in which the former acrylic resin dentures could not provide adequate mastication, but with the use of a soft liner, improved this condition, is shown here.

The patient was a sixty-year-old female who visited our hospital. Her presenting complaint was that she could hardly chew because of severe pain all over the mandibular residual ridge during mastication.

The maxillary ridge was fair, but the mandibular ridge was so severely resorbed that it appeared concave and its covering mucosa was also thin and lacking in elasticity. Some traumatic ulcers were seen on the ridge(Fig. A-4a ～ d). The former complete dentures, which were made six months previously, were satisfactory in terms of the contour, fit and occlusion of the denture. However, when she was asked to occlude, she complained of pain all over the mandibular residual ridge.

Having assessed these conditions, the author tried to line the new lower denture with a soft lining material in order to compensate for the lost thickness of the mucosa and reduce the impact occurring during mastication.

Lining was performed by the indirect method as the thickness of material and lining form can be controlled. A dough type fluorinated soft lining material developed by the author's research group(Kurepeet Dough, Kureha) was used. The material is chemically stable, adheres well to the acrylic resin denture base and can also be easily manipulated(Fig. A-5a, b).

As a result, the pain during mastication diminished, no ulcers were seen on the mucosa and satisfactory progress was obtained. After six months, the surface of the lining material exhibited no contamination, deterioration or abrasion.

Incidentally, as the period of denture wearing becomes prolonged associated with an increase in life span as mentioned previously, the number of cases of severe bone resorption has increased, especially those showing a greatly hollowed-out

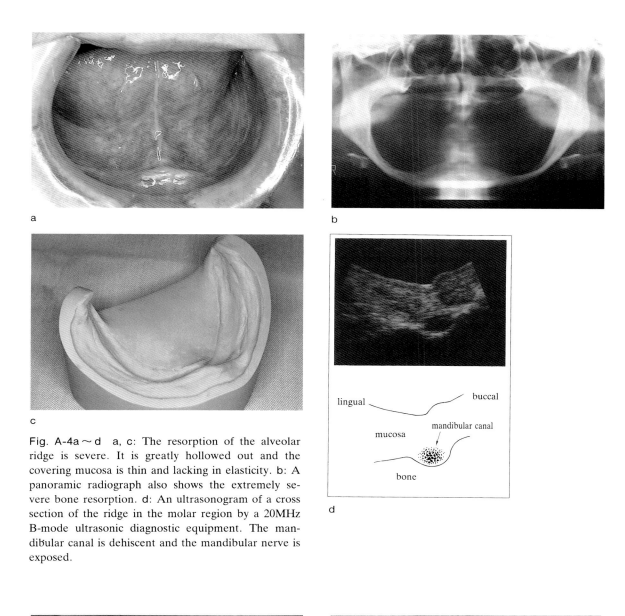

Fig. A-4a ~ d   a, c: The resorption of the alveolar ridge is severe. It is greatly hollowed out and the covering mucosa is thin and lacking in elasticity. b: A panoramic radiograph also shows the extremely severe bone resorption. d: An ultrasonogram of a cross section of the ridge in the molar region by a 20MHz B-mode ultrasonic diagnostic equipment. The mandibular canal is dehiscent and the mandibular nerve is exposed.

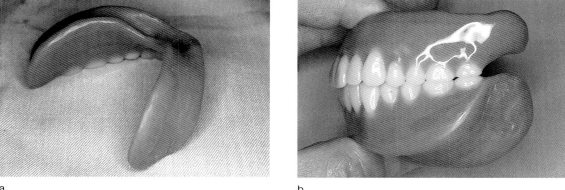

Fig. A-5a, b   a: The mandibular denture lined with a soft liner "Kurepeet Dough". b: New complete dentures.

mandibular ridge, which is probably due to wearing ill-fitting dentures for a long time. The ridge has probably been hollowed out by rolling and pitching of the denture in a similar way as a rock is eroded away by ocean waves. Twenty or thirty years ago when the denture wearing period was not so long, these patterns of resorption were not seen, and the ridge was still flat even when the resorption was severe.

If our lives are progressively prolonged, a steady increase of these kinds of severe resorption can easily be expected. Therefore, the most important point in designing the denture may be how to prevent the resorption of the alveolar ridge including the atrophy of the covering mucosa accompanying the resorption.

4. Kurepeet Dough

This is a dough type soft material. The previous fluorinated soft liner(Kurepeet, Kureha, fluorinated copolymer composed of 50% vinylidene fluoride, 30% chlorotrifluoroethylene and 20% tetraflouroethylene by weight) hardly absorbed water and adhered well to the denture base acrylic resin(Fig. A-6). However, some problems still remained regarding its handling properties and softness. In order to solve these problems, Kurepeet Dough has been developed. In other words, as the new material is provided with plastic properties by mixing with the previous fluoropolymer, a low molecular weight fluorine-containing oligomer, its handling properties are improved and it becomes softer. In addition, in order to improve the strength after lining, the polymerization is induced by introducing a methacrylic radical into the oligomer.

As mentioned above, this dough type lining material possesses plastic properties and polymerizing action, exhibiting good flow during packing and good viscoelasticity after curing due to cross-linking between the molecules.

1) Lining procedure

(1) Invest the waxed denture in a denture flask. After the plaster has set, the wax is eliminated and a separating medium is painted on all surfaces of the stone and plaster (Fig. A-7〜9).

(2) Adapt wax for a spacer on the tissue surface of the cast in the lower half of the flask. Usually, one layer of baseplate wax (1.4 mm in thickness) is used. Depending on the conditions of the underlying mucosa, wax is partially adapted, e.g. on the sharpened alveolar bone or undercut area (Fig. A-11a, b).

(3) Place a polyethylene film over the spacer. Adapt the resin

Fig. A-6   Fluorinated soft liner "Kurepeet Dough". As it is a dough type lining material with plastic properties and polymerizing action, it can flow during packing and after curing, beoming a liner possessing viscoelastic properties.

dough into the upper half of the flask. Place the flask halves in position and close them slowly in a press(Fig. A-12, 13).

(4) Trim the excess resin. Repeat trial packing until no more flash is formed(Fig. A-14).

(5) Assemble the flask with a polyethylene film between the two halves. Place the flask in a press and bench cure the denture for 10 ~ 15 minutes to allow the resin dough to harden. If the lining material is packed while the denture base resin is still soft, the resin dough will be displaced and thus it will be impossible to line the liner evenly(Fig. 15).

(6) Open the flask and remove the spacer. Adapt the lining material dough onto the surface of the hardened denture base resin in the upper half of the flask(Fig. A-16, 17).

(7) Place a polyethylene film on the cast and place the flask halves in position and close them in a press. Repeat trial packing as mentioned above(Fig. A-18, 19).

(8) After no more flash is formed, remove the polyethylene film, close the flask with metal-to-metal contact and place it in a press(Fig. A-20). Then cure the denture as usual (Fig. A-21, 22).

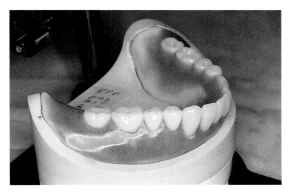

Fig. A-7 After waxing, invest the denture in the flask according to the usual method.

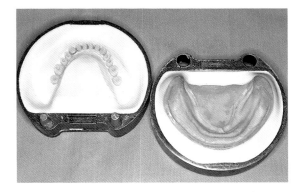

Fig. A-8 After the plaster has set, remove the wax and apply a separating medium.

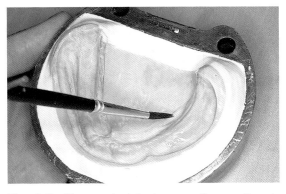

Fig. A-9 The usual alginate separating medium is used for separating Kurepeet Dough from the stone and plaster.

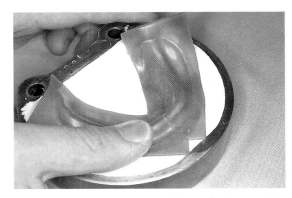

Fig. A-10 Examine the condition of the covering mucosa carefully and control the cushioning effect of the material by varying the thickness of the spacer. Usually, one layer of baseplate wax (1.4 mm in thickness) is used.

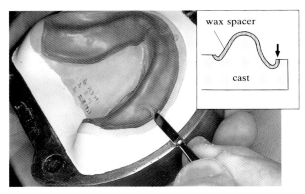

Fig. A-11a, b   As Kurepeet Dough adheres well to the denture base resin, the lining can be extended to the denture border. Cut the wax spacer at the level of the land.

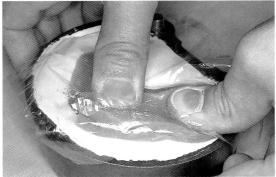

Fig. A-12   Adapt the resin dough in the upper half of the flask as usual. Use denture base resins which are compatible with Kurepeet Dough(Table 3).

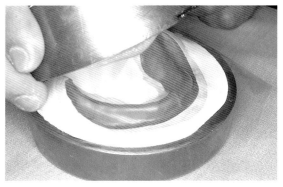

Fig. A-13   Put a polyethylene film over the spacer and cover it with the upper half of the flask packed with the resin dough. Close the flask in a press.

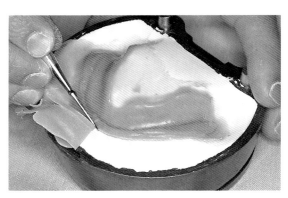

Fig. A-14   Repeat trial packing until no more flash is formed.

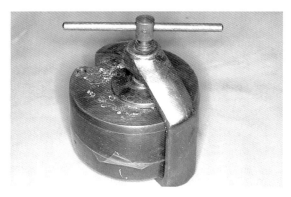

Fig. A-15   Assemble the flask with a polyethylene film, place it in a press and bench cure it for 10～15 minutes.

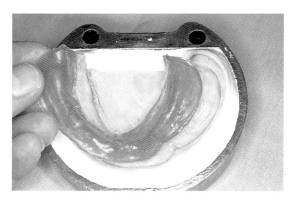

Fig. A-16   Open the flask and remove the spacer wax.

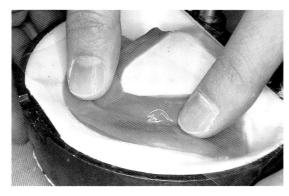

Fig. A-17 Adapt the lining material onto the denture base resin carefully so that voids or bubbles will be minimized at the junction of Kurepeet Dough and the denture base resin. As Kurepeet Dough is somewhat sticky, it is better to apply the supplied separating medium lightly on the fingers.

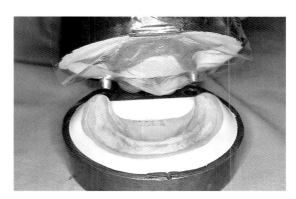

Fig. A-18 Put a polyethylene film on the cast, assemble the flask and close it in a press. Repeat trial packing of the lining material using the same technique used for the denture base resin.

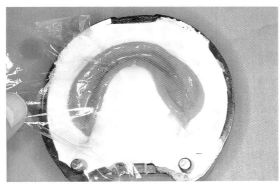

Fig. A-19 The room created by the spacer is filled with Kurepeet Dough. Remove the polyethylene film and check the amount of lining material.

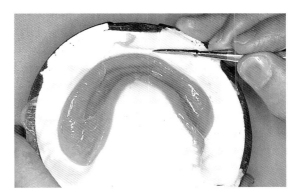

Fig. A-20 Trim the excess material with a knife. Without the polyethylene film, close the flask until metal-to-metal contact is achieved and cure the denture as usual.

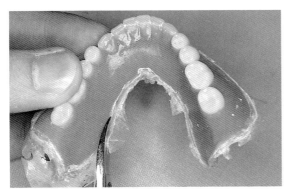

Fig. A-21 After curing, the denture lined with a soft lining material can be easily removed. Remove the flash with scissors.

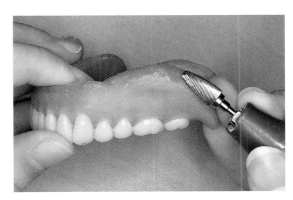

Fig. A-22 Trim the junction of the two materials smoothly with a carbide bur etc..

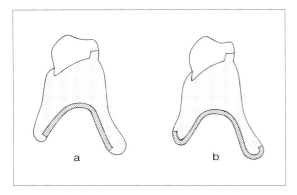

Fig. 23a, b   The lining forms of soft lining materials. If the bond strength of the material to the base resin is low, its margin must be confined within the denture border(a), but a material with a high bond strength can be extended to the denture border(b).

2) Thickness and form

The spacer will be converted to the lining material. Therefore, in order to provide an appropriate cushioning effect to the lining material, one has to control the effect by varying the thickness of the spacer after examining the extent of alveolar bone resorption and the condition of the covering mucosa carefully. Usually, it is sufficient to adapt one layer of baseplate wax(1.4 mm in thickness) all over the ridge of the cast, but if there are sharp alveolar bones or bony prominences, these portions should be covered more thickly. If the soft liner is too thin, it can not exhibit the cushioning effect adequately, but if it is too thick, the rest of the denture base resin will be too thin and fracture of the denture is likely to occur.

Regarding the lining form, with the soft liners such as the silicone lining material, which exhibit a low bond strength, separation can be prevented by confining the margin of the lining material within the denture border[52,53]. However, as Kurepeet Dough adheres well to the denture base resin, it can be extended to the periphery(Fig. A-23). As shown in Fig. A-23a, if the denture border is not lined by the soft lining material, the occlusal load will concentrate on the mucosa beneath the denture border during mastication, causing pain along the periphery.

3) Reasons for surface roughness and measures for prevention

Sometimes roughness or bubbles are seen on the surface of the lining material after curing. This could be mainly due to the difference of polymerization velocity between the Kurepeet Dough and the denture base resins. Namely, if a denture base resin that polymerizes more quickly than Kurepeet Dough is used, as the internal pressure of the resin dough rises due to its expansion when it approaches the curing peak earlier, it will push the Kurepeet Dough out because its polymerization has not yet completed and it is still in a condition where it can easily flow. When Kurepeet Dough later reaches its peak, this displaced portion will not return and will undergo polymerization causing roughness on the lining surface. A similar phenomenon can be seen in the casting procedure of crown and bridge work. Shrinkage porosity also occurs in the area where the casting solidifies last during casting. In order to avoid the displacement of the Kurepeet Dough during polymerization, denture base resins which have a slower polymerization velocity than that of Kurepeet Dough should be used, or the surroundings of the denture periphery should be adequately sealed in the flask.

Table 3   Denture base resins compatible with Kurepeet Dough.

trade names	Manufacturers	trade name	Manufacturers
Acron	GC	New Deburon	Toyo Chemicals
Acrell	Nissin	Lucitone 199	Caulk
α-Resin	Nissin	Meliodent	Bayer
Bio Resin	Shofu	Hirco	Coe

Concerning the former, from the results of an experiment of compatibility between the fluorinated soft material and denture base resins, it has been demonstrated that heat cured denture base resins with a slower polymerization velocity than that of Kurepeet Dough shown in **Table 3** are compatible and can lead to a smooth lining surface[54].

However, even if these appropriate denture base resins are used, roughness may occasionally occur on the lining surface. This may be due to trivial errors of the curing procedure or curing time etc., so in order to always obtain a smooth lining surface an effective measure would be to additionally provide a seal around the denture.

Concerning this sealing method, it has been proven that making a valve filled with the denture base resin dough around the denture during packing is the most effective means

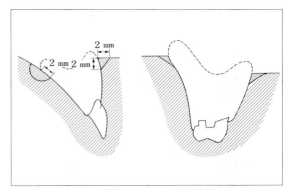

Fig. A-24　Bevel the margins of the mold in the upper half of the flask.

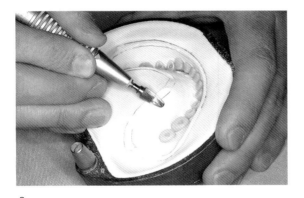

a

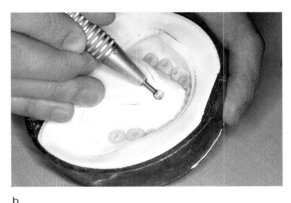

b

Fig. A-25a, b　Bevel the projected margins of the mold(a), and make grooves on the smooth margins of the mold at the anterior lingual and posterior regions of the mandible(b).

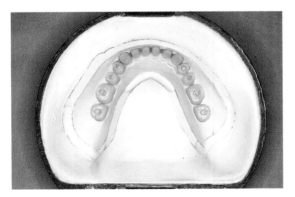

Fig. A-26　Paint the separating medium after bevelling and grooving.

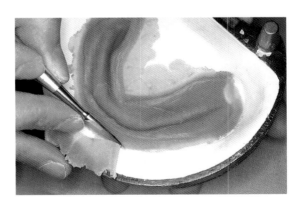

Fig. A-27　After trial packing, eliminate the excess resin outside the bevels and grooves.

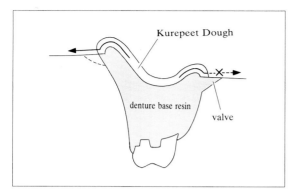

Fig. A-28 The resin dough filling the bevels and grooves will serve as a valve to block the flow of Kurepeet Dough during curing.

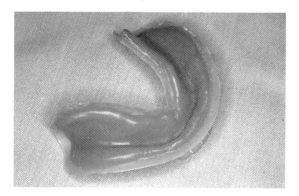

Fig. A-29 The valves remain on the denture after curing. Remove these valves before polishing.

to block the flow of Kurepeet Dough[55](Fig. A-24〜29).

By the way, in the case where the roughness on the lining surface after curing is so great that it cannot be eliminated by polishing, the following measures which may be considered temporary can be used to obtain a smooth surface. After one layer of the rough surface is removed and smoothed, a small amount of Kurepeet Dough should be added to the surface and cured again.

4) Polishing procedure

Even though the polymerization has been performed appropriately and the surface of the lining material is apparently smooth, if the denture is not properly cleaned, the surface will become contaminated in a short period.

Soft liners will crack due to fatigue of the material during prolonged use and will easily become contaminated. But if contamination occurs quickly, the reason for this may be mainly due to the roughness of the surface of the lining material. This roughness is thought to be minute irregularities on the surface of the lining material which was affected by the porous surface of the cast during polymerization.

Therefore, in order to minimize contamination, it is essential to polish the lining surface after polymerization, in a similar manner to the resin denture base. However, as is generally known, it is not easy to polish an elastic material, so a simple polishing method is useful to know. In this method, prior to polishing the lining material after polymerization, the soft lining material is hardened by placing the relined denture in the

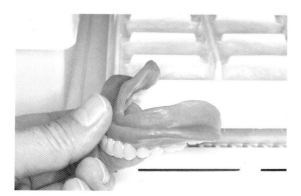

Fig. A-30 Prior to polishing the surface of the lining, the denture is kept in the freezer for 15 minutes to harden the Kurepeet Dough.

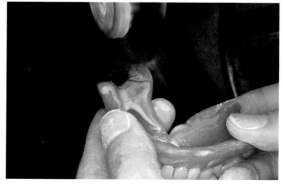

Fig. A-31 Polish the surface using a hard brush and cleanser lightly with a slowly rotating lathe. In order to maintain the hardness of Kurepeet Dough during polishing, occasionally immerse the denture in the iced water.

freezer. This makes it possible to perform the same polishing procedure as is done for the base resin[55,56] (Fig. A-30~33).

When adjusting the lining surface after inserting the denture, pressure points should be eliminated using a carbide bur, and the polishing of the roughened surface after adjustment should then be done using a silicone point for the resin base (Fig. A-34, 35). If the area of elimination due to adjustment is too wide, it would be better to polish the surface with a lathe-mounted brush wheel and flour of pumice after freezing again.

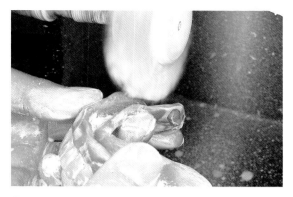

Fig. A-32 Burnishing is done with a soft brush and zinc oxide powder.

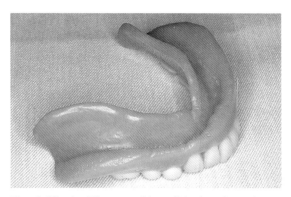
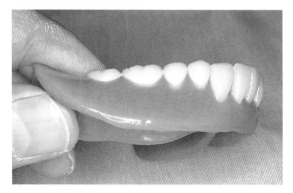

Fig. A-33a, b The smoothly polished surface of the lining. The junction is also smoothly polished.

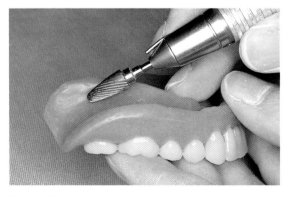
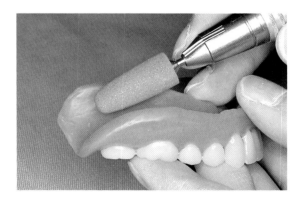

Fig. A-34 Eliminate any pressure areas with a carbide bur.

Fig. A-35 The roughened surface is polished by a silicone point for the resin base.

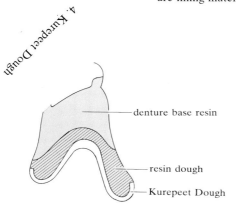

denture base resin

resin dough

Kurepeet Dough

a

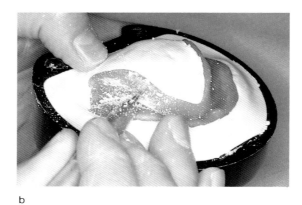

b

Fig. A-36a, b   a: As Kurepeet Dough does not adhere directly to old denture base resin, a layer of resin dough must be placed between them. b: Eliminate the fitting surface of the denture base adequately to obtain a space for both materials.

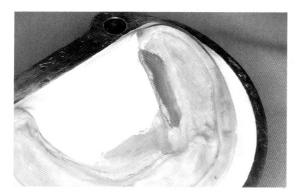

Fig. A-37   Add the necessary amount of wax on the area where the soft lining material is desirable.

5) Relining the denture

The denture should be invested in the flask as usual after the functional impression has been completed. After the plaster has set, the impression material should be removed and then the fitting surface of the denture eliminated. At this time, the space required for Kurepeet Dough and a layer of resin dough ought to be 2-3 mm. Then according to the lining procedure for a new denture, resin and then the Kurepeet Dough should be adapted, and cured. As Kurepeet Dough does not adhere directly to the old denture base resin, new resin dough must be placed between them(Fig. A-36).

6) Partial lining

Add the necessary amount of wax for the spacer only on the part which requires relining with the soft liner. After trial packing for the denture base resin, remove the spacer and adapt Kurepeet Dough in that part. The procedure is similar to that for the fabrication of a new denture(Fig. A-37).

References

1) DuBrul, E. L.: Sicher and DuBrul's Oral anatomy(ed 8). Ishiyaku EuroAmerica Inc., St. Louis, 1988.

2) The academy of denture prosthetics: Glossary of Prosthodontic terms(ed 5), Preston J. D. et al.(ed). The C. V. Mosby Co., St. Louis, 1987.

3) Yazaki, M.: Complete denture prosthesis. Shikagakuho Co., Tokyo, 1935.

4) Okino, S.: Complete denture prosthodontics. Nagasue Publishing Co., Kyoto, 1964.

5) Kamijo, Y.: Oral anatomy 5. Anatom Co., Tokyo, 1969.

6) Wright, C. R., Swartz, W. H., Godwin, W. C.: Mandibular denture stability. The Overbeck Co., Ann Arbor, 1961.

7) Levin, B.: Impressions for complete dentures. Quintessence Publishing Co., Chicago, 1984.

8) Watt, D. M., Macgregor, A. R.: Designing complete dentures. W. B. Saunders Co., Philadelphia, 1976.

9) Hickey, J. C., Zarb, G. A., Bolender, C. L.: Boucher's prosthodontic treatment for edentulous patients(ed 9). The C. V. Mosby Co., St. Louis, 1980.

10) Lye, T. L.: The significance of the fovea palatini in complete denture prosthodontics. J Prosthet Dent, 33: 504-510, 1975.

11) Chen, M.: Reliability of the fovea palatini for determing the posterior border of the maxillary denture. J Prosthet Dent, 43: 133-137, 1980.

12) Jamieson, C. H.: A modern concept of complete dentures. J Prosthet Dent, 6: 582-592, 1956.

13) Hartono, R.: The occlusal plane in relation to facial types. J Prosthet Dent, 17: 549-559, 1967.

14) Uehara, J. et al.: A roentgenographic cephalometric study on naso-auricular line. Kanagawa Sigaku, 5: 1-7, 1970.

15) Augusburger, R. H.: Occlusal plane relation to facial type. J Prosthet Dent, 3: 755-770, 1953.

16) Hayakawa, I. et al.: A roentgenographic cephalometric study on occlusal plane. J Jpn Prosthodont Soc, 19: 294-298, 1975.

17) Hayakawa, I. et al.: A roentgenographic cephalometric study on vertical dimension(Prediction for vertical dimension). J Jpn Prosthodont Soc, 20: 186-192, 1976.

18) Hayakawa, I. et al.: Prediction formulae for the vertical dimension and the vertical dimension indicator. Dental Outlook, 67: 813-818, 1986.

19) Hayashi, T.: On the occlusion of complete dentures. Dental Review, 376: 97-110, 1974.

20) Nemoto, K.: A study on the three dimenisonal range of the mandibular movement at the incision inferius. J Jpn Prosthodont Soc, 6: 1-40, 1962.

21) Posselt, U.: Physiology of occlusion and rehabilitaion(ed 2). Blackwell Scientific Publications, London, 1968.

22) Lin, C.: A clinical study of horizontal maxillomandibular relation records in the edentulous. J Jpn Prosthodont Soc, 26: 340-360, 1982.

23) Ishihara, T. et al.: Movements of the mandible. Dental Outlook, 31: 29-40, 1968.

24) Hayashi, T. et al.: Complete denture prosthodontics(ed 3). Ishiyaku Publishing Co., Tokyo, 1993.

25) Gysi, A.: Practical application of research results in denture construction. J Am Dent Assoc, 16: 199-223, 1929.

26) Rinaldi, P., Sharry, J.: Tongue force and fatigue in adults. J Prosthet Dent, 13: 857-865, 1963.

27) Tsubone, M., Toyoda, S.: Clinical morphology of complete dentures. Ishiyaku Publishing Co., Tokyo, 1978.

28) Schiffman, P.: Relation of the maxillary canines to the incisive papilla. J Prosthet Dent, 14: 469-472, 1964.

29) Pound, E.: Recapturing esthetic tooth position in the edentulous patient. J Am Dent Assoc, 55: 181-191, 1957.

30) Ortman, H. R., Ortman, L. F.:(Arrangement of the posterior teeth) Essentials of complete denture prosthodontics. W. B. Sounders Co., Philadelphia, 1979.

31) Fish, E. W.: Principles of full denture prosthesis(ed 4): Staples Press Co., London, 1948.

32) Schultz, A. W.: Comfort and chewing efficiency in dentures. J Prosthet Dent, 1: 38-48, 1951.

33) Brill, N. et al.: The role of exteroceptors in denture retention. J Prosthet Dent, 9: 761-768, 1959.

34) Matsumoto, N.: A chronological study on the form of clinical tooth crown. J Stomatol Soc Jpn, 32: 108-136, 1965.

35) Lott, F. et al.: Flange technique, an anatomic and physiologic approach to increased retention, comfort, and appearance of dentures. J Prosthet Dent, 16: 394-413, 1966.

36) Beresin, V. E., Schiesser, F. J.: The neutral zone in complete dentures. The C. V. Mosby Co., Saint Louis, 1973.

37) Lammie, G. A.: Aging changes and the complete lower denture. J Prosthet Dent, 6: 450-464, 1954.

38) Ai, M.: A study of the masticatory movement at the incision inferius. J Jpn Posthodont Soc, 6: 164-200, 1962.

39) Department of Prosthodontics, School of Dentistry, Oregon Health Sciences University: Clinical syllabus for complete dentures(1991-92). Oregon Health Sciences University, Oregon, 1991.

40) Hayakawa, I.: Impressions for complete dentures using a new silicone impression material; One-step border molding technique. The Quintessence, 17: 45-51, 1998.

41) Phillips, R. W.: Skinner's science of dental materials(ed 7). W. B. Saunders Co., Philadelphia, 1973.

42) Morii, K. et al.: Microbiological aspects of filth on acrylic soft denture liners. J Jpn Prosthodont Soc, 22: 679-683, 1978.

43) Gibbons, P.: Clinical and bacteriological findings in patients wearing Silastic 390 soft liner. J Mich S Dent A, 47: 64-67, 1965.

44) Hayakawa, I. et al.: Development of soft denture liner(dough-type) of fluoroetylene copolymer. J Jpn Prosthodont Soc, 30: 321-325, 1986.

45) Tsuru, H.: Denture construction with the resilient denture liner "Molteno" using a new adhesive technique. Dental Technology, 18: 445-452, 1990.

46) Hayakawa, I. et al.: The creap behavior of denture-supporting tissues and soft lining materials. Int J Prosthodont, 7: 339-347, 1994.

47) Matsumoto, T. et al.: Study on a light cured soft lining material. International congress on dental materials, transactions.: 437-438, 1989.

48) Lammie, G. A.: A preliminary report on resilient denture plastics. J Prosthet Dent, 8: 411-424, 1958.

49) Akiyoshi, R.: A complete denture provided peripheral seal with resilient material, a case report. Practice in Prosthodontics, 3: 175-179, 1970.

50) Hayakawa, I. et al.: Development of the coating material for tissue conditioner. J Jpn Prosthodont Soc, 27: 780-783, 1983.

51) Hayakawa, I. et al.: The effect of a fluorinated copolymer coating agent on tissue conditioners. Int J Prosthodont, 10: 44-48, 1997.

52) Storer, R.: Resilient denture base materials part 2, clinical trial. Br Dent J, 113: 231-239, 1962.

53) Sauer, J. L.: A clinical evaluation of Silastic 390 as a lining material for dentures. J Prosthet Dent, 16: 650-660, 1966.

54) Hayakawa, I. et al.: Compatibility between dough-type fluoropolymer soft liner "Kurepeet Dough" and denture base resins and coating effect of a coating material. J J Dent Mater, 6: 894-898, 1987.

55) Hirano, S. et al.: Clinical application of soft denture liner (Kurepeet Dough). DE, 105: 2-7, 1993.

56) Hayakawa, I. et al.: Pre-packing treatment and polishing of fluorinated soft lining material "Kurepeet Dough". QDT, 17: 108-110, 1992.

Index